Your Hearing Loss

How to Break the Sound Barrier

Consultants:

John R. Cochran, Ph.D.
Kearney State College

Donal H. Morgan, M.D.
Southwest Nebraska Medical Cente

Illustrations:

Karen Helleberg

Your Hearing Loss

How to Break the Sound Barrier

Marilyn M. Helleberg, M.S.

Nelson-Hall nh Chicago

Library of Congress Cataloging in Publication Data

Helleberg, Marilyn M.
Your Hearing Loss.

Bibliography: p.
Includes index.
1. Hearing disorders. 2. Deaf — Rehabilitation.
I. Title.
RF290.H44 617.8 78-8663
ISBN 0-88229-341-9

Reprinted 1980

Manufactured in the United States of America

10 9 8 7 6 5 4 3 2

To Rex, my co-pilot

Contents

Acknowledgments

This book would not have been possible without the contributions of many interested individuals.

My sincere thanks to William Steubing of Nelson-Hall, who first contacted me about writing the book, and to the other Nelson-Hall editors who have worked with me to make the book a reality.

To John R. Cochran, Ph.D., and Donal H. Morgan, M.D., whose professional input and careful analysis of the manuscript contributed valuable suggestions for improvement, I am deeply grateful.

The thorough reading of the manuscript by a severely hard-of-hearing friend, Beverly Thomas, provided a worthwhile testing ground for the material it contains.

To Joyce Roberts goes the credit for the tedious job of typing the several drafts of the manuscript.

I'd also like to thank the following publishers for allowing me to quote from a wide variety of sources: Alexander Graham Bell Association for the Deaf; Channing L. Bete Co., Inc.; Better Hearing Institute; J & A Churchill Publishers; Council of Better Business Bureaus, Inc.; Guideposts Magazine; Holt, Rinehart and Winston; Journal of Rehabilitation of the Deaf; J.B. Lippincott Co.; Maico Audiological Library; National Association of the Deaf; Prentice-Hall, Inc.; The Strode Publishers; Charles C. Thomas Publisher; Volta Bureau; and Joseph Wiedenmayer.

Finally, my special appreciation goes to my husband, Rex Helleberg, and to two members of his architectural staff, Fred Lohmann and Loel Kugler, for their help with the phonetic placement diagrams, and to my daughter, Karen, for her interest-catching illustrations.

Foreword

Your Hearing Loss: How to "Break the Sound Barrier," seems to me to be a very complete work for the person who has developed a hearing loss and is concerned about his future.

The book is factual, and I think it will be recommended by many doctors for their patients with hearing losses. It is readily understood, and I feel that the layman will find within its pages many answers to his questions about hearing loss.

I have never found a book of this type that is so complete in its explanations for the hearing handicapped. It should provide help and encouragement to people with all kinds of hearing loss.

Donal H. Morgan, M.D.
Southwest Nebraska Medical Center
McCook, Nebraska

Introduction

"Eh?" the old fellow says, with his hand cupped behind his ear. And everyone laughs. Or do they? Millions of people—those who have a handicapping degree of hearing loss—do not laugh. To experience confusion, embarrassment, job restrictions, and social isolation day after day is not funny.

Most likely, you have heard the old saying, "What you don't know won't hurt you." Many persons comfort themselves in their ignorance, or excuse their lack of initiative, with this saying. The fact is, however, that what you don't know about hearing loss can hurt you in a great many ways. It can increase tension, suspicion, resentment, depression, and irritability. It can keep you from a promotion you deserve, from conversations with friends, from normal give and take in and out of the home, from full participation in life. That fuller participation is possible is the sure conviction of the author and the recurring theme in this book.

From professional training, from personal experience in her own family, and with a warm, genuine approach, Marilyn Helleberg has put together here a sort of guide book on hearing loss. This book is for the average person who doesn't want a lot of eighty-five cent words but does want solid facts, simply and clearly stated. With humor, with kindness, with sensitivity and insight, the reader is led to a clearer understanding of why Johnny can't hear, why Grandpa says "Eh," why wife is getting cranky, or why you are beginning to think that no one talks clearly anymore. This understanding is developed through a discussion of causes of hearing loss; normal, to-be-expected emotional reactions to loss; remedial measures that are often helpful; the use, functions, and values of hearing aids; how lipreading training may help; recent discoveries and developments that offer new hope; suggestions for further reading on special topics; and directions for finding skilled help for special needs.

Alfred Noyes said, "Each new grain of truth is packed, like radium, with whole new worlds of light." This book can bring many new grains of truth that can shed greater light upon your understanding of hearing loss and of the often special world of the hearing impaired. No one wants to feel that he is somehow a curiosity to others, or an object of pity, humor, or rejection. So, take up this little volume with a sense of discovery, challenge, and responsibility. You'll be glad you did. And, so will others.

John R. Cochran, Ph.D.
Director, Speech and Hearing Clinic
Kearney State College
Kearney, Nebraska

Letter to You—My Reader

This is a heart-level book. I couldn't have written it any other way, because I've never been able to be completely impersonal in working with the hard of hearing. Maybe that's because my own husband, Rex, has a hearing loss. Since you and I are going to be spending some time together, I'd like to have you think of me as a friend, and of this book as your personal guide to a better understanding of your hearing problem. It is sprinkled with personal experiences, because this is my way of identifying with your problem.

In the pages that follow, I've put into everyday language many of the facts about hearing loss that I have taught my college students in audiology and aural rehabilitation classes. Then I've taken therapy techniques that have *worked* for me as a speech and hearing clinician and adapted them so that you can use them at home to improve your ability to understand speech, to lipread, and to speak more clearly, and to cope with the social and emotional problems your hearing loss causes.

I've tried to write the book in a way that will make it useful to adults with various degrees and types of hearing impairments. For this reason, you'll probably find a section, here and there, that doesn't apply directly to you. The question-answer presentation should make it easy for you to zero in on those aspects that are of greatest concern to you. Still, Beverly (my hard-of-hearing friend who has read the manuscript) said she was glad she read every word, because it helped her to understand *other* types of hearing loss, and it unearthed for her some interesting contrasts and similarities.

But what's the purpose of all this? Maybe this little anecdote from my own life will suggest the answer to that question.

Several years ago, I decided I wanted to become an airplane pilot, but I walked away from my first flying lesson, reeking of insecurity and self-doubt.

"I'll never learn to fly," I moaned. "I'm afraid of heights, I have a fear of falling, and I can't understand that jumbled mumbling coming over the radio from the control tower. I give up!"

But the next week, with Rex's encouragement, I started 'ground school' and began to learn about what makes an airplane fly, what signals trouble, how to interpret those garbled radio cues, what to do when I lose my way, and how to tune in to all those people on the ground who are there to help me. I found out that the more you know about something, the less threatening it is.

We all feel threatened by things we don't fully understand, and hearing loss is no exception. To the extent that you don't understand your hearing problem, it controls you. But the more you can learn about it, the more ready you'll be to take over the controls and aim your nose into the wind.

Fear of the unknown made me say, "I'll never learn to fly." Fear of the unknown makes many hard-of-hearing adults feel like giving up. But the day I got my private pilot's license, I realized that fear could be another word for challenge. I hope this book will change fear to challenge in your mind and heart.

Our course is plotted, the runway is clear, visibility is good. Let's break the sound barrier!

Part One

What do I need to know about hearing loss?

1

Can I lead a fulfilling life in spite of my hearing loss?

One spring, when I was about ten years old, I was planning to enter a city-wide kite-flying contest. Kites were a big thing in McCook, Nebraska, in the thirties. I'd been saving my dime-a-week allowance to buy a beautiful Chinese dragon kite I'd seen in a hardware store downtown. A few days before the contest, I put my ten dimes in my purse, placed the purse in my bike basket, and pedaled to town. When I parked my bike in front of the store and reached into the basket for my purse, I discovered, to my horror, that the ride had jiggled loose the clasp on my purse. Gasping, I grabbed the purse and looked inside. One, two, three dimes! I needed ten! It would be *seven more weeks* before I'd again have enough money to buy my kite, and by that time, it would be too late. Maybe I could find the lost dimes! I walked my bike home, inching along, searching, but I only found one more dime. When I walked in the door with tears streaming down my face and told my mother what had happened, she put her arms around me and said, "You've lost something that was very valuable to you. Let's see, now, what can you do about it? You can drop out of the contest and put the three dimes back in your drawer and forget about them. Or you can take what you have left and figure out a way to stay in the contest. It's up to you."

I dried my eyes on the edge of my sleeve, and the next day my father and I went to the lumber yard and bought some white pine sticks and two balls of string with my three dimes. (Things were cheaper in those days!) That night, we built a box kite out of the sticks and some brown wrapping paper, and I painted bright red dragons on all four sides. It didn't look as good as the store kite, but to me it was beautiful.

I'd like to be able to say that I won first place in the kite-flying contest, but I didn't. My kite wobbled, and I couldn't get it up very high. But I did get honorable mention for the "most creative homemade kite." I got something else, too. I got a mighty tool for successful living that would last me the rest of my life. *That's* winning.

You've lost your hearing—or part of it. That's one of the most valuable things that anyone could ever lose. What do you have left? Four other senses, *some* hearing that's still usable (almost no one is totally deaf), your native intelligence, lots of people who want to help you, and, I hope, a determination to stay in the contest. That's all you need. Even though your hearing is impaired, you don't have to settle for less than a full measure of life, if you'll take what you have left out of the drawer and use it. Let's begin by answering some of your questions about hearing loss.

How many hard-of-hearing people are there? If you have impaired hearing, you are a member of a surprisingly large fraternity. There are more people in the United States with less-than-normal hearing than there are people living in the whole state of Ohio; more than the entire student population of all U.S. colleges and universities; more than the total number of United States government employees. The number of Americans with hearing losses is five times greater than the population of Chicago, eight times greater than the number of marriages performed in 1973, fifteen times greater than the national membership of the Beneficent and Protective Order of Elks. According to the U.S. Department of Health, Education, and Welfare, impaired hearing is the nation's number one physical disability. Nearly ten percent of the population of every city and village in the world has defective hearing to some degree. This includes approximately 15 million Americans. It means that, in a crowd of 100 people, there are 10 who could touch your hand and say, "I *know* how you feel. I have a hearing problem, too."

The proportion of people with a hearing disorder is almost certainly increasing because doctors are learning how to save more and more of the babies who have difficult births or are born prematurely. Some of these babies have defective hearing. Also, more and more of us are being exposed to extremely loud noise, and more and more of us are living into the older ages during which impaired hearing has always been most common.

But why am I not aware of all these other people who have hearing losses? For one thing, many of them function quite normally in society. Often, there is no visible sign that would indicate that an individual is hard of hearing. Modern hearing aids are often quite inconspicuous, and more and more people with impaired hearing have sought and received help in speechreading, auditory training, and speech conservation, so that they can still communicate quite well. Unfortunately, there are also many people with slightly defective hearing who refuse to admit that they have a problem.

Well, as long as they're able to conceal the fact that they have a loss, what harm is there in that? In the first place, they may not be concealing it as well as they think they are. Bluffing is a defense mechanism. A person who is trying to deny the fact that he has a hearing problem often pretends to understand when he really doesn't. This may cause him to make inappropriate replies, or he may fall into the 'yes' and 'no' habit of responding.

How is this interpreted by the person who's talking? He may assume that the 'bluffer' is just refusing to listen, so the speaker thinks, "I must be boring him," or "Maybe he's angry with me," or "This guy sure is stuck-up." In any case, he soon ends the lame conversation, and the hard-of-hearing person may have alienated a good friend or lost the chance for making a new one. Worse yet, if the speaker doesn't know his listener very well, he may assume that he's just not very bright, or that he's getting senile, or make some other such negative judgment.

Aside from the social aspects, is there anything else wrong with trying to conceal a hearing problem? Yes. Your hearing defect may be correctable by medical, surgical, or mechanical means. But all of the recent advances in medicine and technology will not help you if you refuse to seek that help. In a booklet published by Better Hearing Institute, Nanette Fabray, star of theater, musical comedy, television and motion pictures, says,

> I was born with a progressive deafness. Years ago, while starring in "Bloomer Girl," I had reason to soon expect total deafness. I tried to conceal my handicap, and desperately withdrew into myself, as people often do with hearing problems. Thanks to corrective surgery, and continued use of hearing aids, I came back from the edge of early retirement. Hopefully, my own experience will encourage others to seek qualified help and advice. Hiding the problem hides the cure.[1]

Are all hearing losses correctable, then? Physically, no. If your hearing impairment is caused by a problem in the outer or middle ear, it may respond to medical or surgical treatment. Losses of this type are called *conductive.* (See Chapter 3.) Chapter 5 explains some of the treatments available for conductive losses. But if the problem is sensori-neural (that is, if it is caused by a defect in the inner ear or in the nerve pathway to the brain), it is probably not medically correctable. (See Chapters 4 and 5.)

Then if I have a "nerve loss," why should I seek help? In the first place, there is no way you can know for sure whether your problem is conductive or sensori-neural and whether or not it is correctable unless you have a complete medical and audiological evaluation.

You mean I should see my family doctor? That's the first step. He'll give you a thorough examination to see if there's a clear-cut physical problem affecting your hearing. He may decide to refer you to an otologist.

What's an otologist? An otologist is a medical doctor who specializes in diseases of the ear. Otology is one division of the ear-nose-and-throat field of medicine. An otologist diagnoses diseases of the ear, specifies causes of hearing impairment, and treats physical defects of the auditory mechanism. He may have an audiologist assist him in his evaluation; or your family doctor may refer you directly to an audiologist.

What does an audiologist do? An audiologist is a person with a master's degree or a Ph.D. in audiology who specializes in hearing assessment, or testing, and in the rehabilitation of hard-of-hearing persons. Although some hearing-aid dealers call themselves "audiologists," this title should be reserved for those who have at least a master's degree in audiology. When I use the term audiologist in this book, I am referring only to those professional people who have such degrees. Your family doctor, the otologist, or the audiologist may refer you to a hearing aid dealer.

Why can't I just go see the hearing-aid dealer on my own and save all of those professional fees? It is always advisable to see a doctor first, in order to rule out correctable medical problems that may be causing, or intensifying, your hearing problem. An audiologist may want to give you special diagnostic tests that the hearing-aid dealer may not have the training or equipment to perform. Then too, many professional audiologists keep an assortment of various brands and types of hearing aids, so that they can help you choose the best one for your personal needs. An audiologist may also provide you with rehabilitation therapy or refer you to a speech pathologist for training in speechreading, auditory training, and speech therapy. You will still buy your hearing aid from a hearing-aid dealer, who can also provide you with other mechanical helps that will make your life easier. (See Chapters 8 and 15.)

I can see the need for medical and audiological evaluation if you think you have a hearing problem, but what signs are there that indicate you should seek this kind of assessment? The early symptoms of hearing loss are often very easy to overlook. Yet, the earlier a hearing problem is discovered, the greater the chances are for handling it successfully. Without treatment, temporary hearing impairments can become permanent ones, mild losses can develop into severe handicaps, and losses in a few frequencies may extend into all frequencies.

If I had checked my purse on the way to the store to buy the kite, I could have snapped it shut and saved some of those dimes, if not all of them.

Even in cases where nothing can be done to improve hearing acuity or to keep it from deteriorating further, early detection is crucial. Everyone has noticed that the speech of a person who is losing his hearing is likely to change for the worse. This regression can be stopped or held in check if it's discovered early enough. With prompt special help in speechreading and auditory training, the person who is losing his hearing can acquire skills that will help him to compensate, while he still has enough hearing to learn them easily. Ask yourself these questions:

1. Do people seem to be mumbling a lot?
2. Are you often surprised when someone calls you to the phone, because you didn't hear it ring?
3. Do you sometimes have trouble *understanding* people, even though you hear their voices clearly?
4. Does noise seem to bother you more than it used to?
5. Are you often startled when someone walks up behind you?
6. Do members of your family walk into the room when you're watching TV and turn the volume down?
7. Do you find yourself saying "What?" or asking people to repeat what they've said?
8. Do people sometimes tell *you* to "tone down your voice a little"?
9. OR, do they ask you to "speak up"?
10. Are people starting to tell *you* to "stop mumbling"?
11. Are you getting so you avoid talking on the telephone unless it's quite necessary?

12. Do you find that you hear better when you can see the speaker's face?

13. Is it getting harder for you to carry on a conversation in a noisy restaurant?

14. OR, do you actually seem to hear better in noisy places?

15. Do you have to strain to follow a lecturer's train of thought or the minister's sermon?

16. Do you have trouble with frequent "ringing in the ears"?

A yes answer to any of these questions *might* be a warning signal to alert you to the early stages of hearing loss. Some of these symptoms, such as numbers 8–9 and 13–14, are direct opposites, but this is because they signal different *types* of hearing loss. Of course, one yes answer doesn't necessarily mean that you *have* a hearing problem. (Maybe your wife really *does* mumble!) But if you have more than one affirmative answer, the probability becomes greater. You should definitely have an evaluation.

But what if I can't afford it? There is only one answer to that question. You can't afford *not* to. If medical and audiological assessment would put a *serious* strain on your budget, there are agencies that will help you. (See Chapter 14.)

Is hearing loss linked with mental deterioration? Fred, a sixty-five-year-old retired college teacher, was living with his daughter and her family. Sue was the first to notice the change in her father. He seemed to be losing some of his alertness and sharp wit. He often had a blank or puzzled look on his face during family conversations. When the children asked him questions, his answers were frequently inappropriate or way off the subject. "Dad's getting senile," she told her husband one day, when the older man got a telephone message all mixed up. Fortunately, her husband suggested that she get her father an appointment with the doctor. When Fred told the doctor about the ringing in his ears, the medical man recommended a hearing evaluation. The audiologist found that Fred had a high-frequency hearing loss that caused him to miss most of the consonant sounds in people's speech. With the help of a hearing aid and aural rehabilitation therapy, Fred soon became as alert as ever. Fred is one of the lucky ones. A distressingly large number of people, particularly those in the older age brackets, are considered to be senile or mentally incompetent because they have undetected hearing losses.

Why do so many people associate deafness with lack of mental

ability? Part of it goes back to that unfortunate term *deaf and dumb,* which originated in medieval times. In the beginning, the term *dumb* simply meant "without speech." Because we learn to speak by imitating what we hear, persons who were born deaf did not develop language. Since deafness and the inability to speak went together, people just assumed that they both resulted from mental defectiveness, instead of realizing that lack of hearing was the *cause* of the muteness. It is probable that our present-day slang use of the word *dumb* as a synonym for *stupid* has its roots in the supposed mental incapacity of the deaf. Today, of course, many congenitally deaf children learn to speak through touch, sight, and the sense of movement, or to communicate through the use of manual alphabets and the language of signs; so they are able to demonstrate the fact that their intelligence is not impaired. The stigma is going! More and more, people are being educated to the fact that deafness is nothing to be ashamed of. Many prominent people with hearing losses are coming forth to tell of their experiences in rising above the problems of deafness and impaired hearing. These success stories will certainly provide encouragement to millions of Americans. We'll hear from some of these people later on in this chapter.

But aren't some hearing-impaired people also mentally deficient? Sure. So are some normally hearing people. As Dr. McCay Vernon points out, "The intelligence of deaf and hard-of-hearing persons has been extensively studied since the advent of IQ tests in the early 1900s. Based on this research, representing approximately fifty independently conducted investigations, it is evident that the deaf and hard-of-hearing population has essentially the same distribution of intelligence as the general population."[2]

The hearing impaired are finally breaking through that dark cloud that the ignorance of normally hearing people has so long held over their heads. This is sunrise news. Of course, *you've* known the truth all along, but now the public is waking up to the facts. Good morning!

In addition to being equally intelligent, the deaf and hard of hearing also compare favorably with normally hearing people in the day-to-day business of living. Their work habits are good, employers who hire them like them, they can excel in sports, have happy marriages, be good parents, and they are better drivers than people with normal hearing. Let's talk about these capabilities, one at a time.

You mean hearing loss doesn't hinder driving ability? That's right. In fact, studies of the driving records of the deaf show that they are the world's safest motorists. Deaf drivers are now granted driver's licenses in all states.

Why do deaf drivers have fewer accidents? For one thing, their hearing losses have taught them to be both alert and cautious. They have developed their powers of observation to a high degree and have learned to focus attentively on whatever they are doing. They are not distracted by conversation and outside noises, and, perhaps most important, they are eager to prove their own capability, and driving gives them a chance to do just that.

Isn't poor hearing a handicap in sports? It doesn't have to be. "Larry Brown, star halfback of the Washington Redskins, was Pro Football's Most Valuable Player in 1972." Brown says:

> The great Vince Lombardi once noticed that I moved well on plays from one side of the line, but that I hesitated in getting out from the other side. "Are you hard of hearing, Larry?" he asked. I admitted that my one ear had a hearing loss, and Lombardi encouraged me to have it corrected. Now, a built-in hearing aid in my helmet enables me to hear all calls clearly. I now move out quickly on both sides. It makes all the difference in the world.[3]

"Tony Zale, former two-time middleweight champion of the world in 1940–48, is currently head coach and coordinator for the Chicago Park District. His hearing loss is the result of an accident." Zale says:

> It didn't take too much prodding for me to get help, and I'm thankful I did. Most hard-of-hearing people could be helped if they would only admit their problem and take steps to correct it.[4]

What about marriage for the aurally handicapped? Deaf and hard-of-hearing people need to be reassured of the fact that they can find happiness in marriage. A high percentage of hearing-impaired people do marry. Hearing loss itself causes them to be deeply attuned to their own inner feelings and to those of their partner, which is an important factor in all good marriages. Those who have normally hearing mates will find the suggestions in Chapter 15 helpful for establishing and maintaining good relationships. Intermarriage of deaf men and women is very common. Such a marriage provides a feeling of security, common interests, and mutual understanding, bringing about a very close relationship. Although deafness of both partners may present some problems with regard to children, these are not insurmountable.

Is it wise for people with defective hearing to have children? Some types of hearing impairment are inherited, and some are not. When deafness "runs in the family," a geneticist, who takes a complete family history, can advise a couple as to the risk of having a hearing-handicapped child. A list of genetic counseling centers appears on page 2 of *Counseling and Medical Genetics* by Sheldon Reed, Ph.D. Your own doctor may know of a genetic counselor in your area. If such a counselor advises you against having a child of your own, you may want to adopt one. With a few extra precautions and the help of signaling devices around the home (see Chapter 15), you can be a successful parent. If you and your spouse are both deaf but your child has normal hearing, you will need to realize the urgent importance of seeing to it that your child has plenty of speech stimulation for normal language development. Maybe a grandparent or aunt can live in, at least during the preschool years, to help provide this vital language input.

On the subject of having children, I can't resist telling you a little story that was told to me by the husband of one of my severely hard-of-hearing friends. He says that the reason they have so many children is that, every night at bedtime, he says to his wife , "Do you want to read, or go to sleep or what? She always answers, "WHAT!" (Hmm. Well, this *is* a book for adults.)

But what about my career? What kinds of jobs are available for the hearing handicapped? There is no need to provide a list of job opportunities, because there are very few fields in which the hard of hearing cannot excel if they have enough deep-down determination and a solid belief in their own abilities. Joseph Wiedenmayer was born hard of hearing and, except by using the most powerful hearing aid, cannot even hear the sound of voices. He makes this valid observation: "All men were not created equal—physically. They become equal or superior to others if they try hard enough and long enough to overcome their handicap." Mr. Wiedenmayer goes on to say that "it is not the extent of our handicap but rather the extent of our ability to overcome it that is important." Burn these words into the grain of your mind and heart, and repeat them to yourself the next time you're tempted to say, "I can't because I'm hard of hearing."

What would have happened if Ludwig van Beethoven, Sir Joshua Reynolds, or Thomas Edison had said, "I can't"? They are just a few of the many overcomers who have made history in spite of their hearing losses. You can make your life count, too! If you have a hearing loss (or think you might) but have been reluctant to seek help, here are some comments from a few of today's prominent hard-of-hearing Americans who are saying, "I can."

"VANCE HARTKE, U.S. SENATOR: 'My hearing was fading for years. At last, I decided to do something about it. My doctor suggested one of those remarkable operations, and I was soon back 'on the air' with much improvement.

'My hearing began to fade again, but with two subsequent operations and the temporary use of a hearing aid, I was able to prevent permanent deterioration.'"[5]

"NORM CROSBY, T.V. AND NIGHTCLUB COMEDIAN: 'I have a hearing loss. I make no bones about the fact that I wear a hearing aid—and that it helps me immeasurably. I speak about it on T.V. and radio talk shows, at meetings, every chance I get. I am heartened that a growing number of hard-of-hearing public figures now talk openly about their handicap—and how they overcame it.'"

"DENCY DAY, AGE 16, RODEO QUEEN: 'I became hard of hearing when I was about a year old. My parents noticed that my two sisters and I weren't learning to speak as we should. They took us to a well-known doctor and found out we all had severe hearing losses. We learned to talk with the use of hearing aids and help from speech therapists. Now I'm a junior in high school. I enjoy basketball and playing in the band. I have won many buckles and trophies in 4-H and high school rodeos, but the thrill of my life came when I was crowned Miss Faith Stock Show Rodeo Queen.

'Without help I would never have learned to speak, so hopefully my experience will help many others with hearing problems.'"[7]

"SOL LESSER, NOTED HOLLYWOOD FILM PRODUCER: 'Deafness is an unseen physical impairment that makes many of us unable to carry on our basic work through speech and response. I wear a hearing aid without equivocation or embarrassment, and am now at ease with friends and associates, am able to enjoy the theater, be at my best at social events and meetings.'"

"FREDERIC MARCH, ACADEMY-AWARD-WINNING ACTOR: 'Because verbal communication is so vital to me, I value good hearing which, thanks to correction of a hearing loss, I continue to enjoy. My own experience convinces me that others missing a part of life because of hearing defects can also be helped. I urge them to see their doctor and to have their hearing tested as soon as possible.'"[9]

"DALE MILFORD, MEMBER OF THE U.S. HOUSE OF REPRESENTATIVES: 'I have probably suffered a very gradual hearing loss over the years due to the high levels of noise I have been exposed to as a professional aviator during most of my adult life. I just hope anyone else who might suspect a gradual hearing loss will take the time and trouble—as I finally did—to find out. And if there is a deficiency which is correctable, have it corrected.'"[10]

"FRED O'GREEN, PRESIDENT OF LITTON INDUSTRIES, one of the nation's leading corporations: 'My hearing loss has not hampered my effectiveness because I did something about it. I had my hearing tested and corrected my problem with a hearing aid.

'Time is the enemy of remedial help for a hearing loss. The longer one waits, the more difficult the recovery. This is why I urge everyone I know with a hearing problem to get an immediate medical checkup.'"[11]

"JOHNNIE RAY, INTERNATIONALLY ACCLAIMED SINGER: 'My hearing problem started around the sixth grade. Later a high school teacher told my parents I was mentally retarded—and suggested I should be put in some sort of an institution. Through those years I became withdrawn and lonely and didn't communicate with anyone. But my parents took me to a doctor and found out I had a serious hearing loss. They got me my first hearing aid at fifteen. I rediscovered the world and was on my way.'"[12]

"GEORGE C. WALLACE, GOVERNOR OF ALABAMA: 'Many people feel there is a terrible stigma attached to losing one's hearing, to wearing a hearing aid. I was no exception. But because I value good hearing, I am no longer a reluctant hearing-aid wearer. Many others with untreated hearing problems can similarly get help, either medically or by amplification.'"[13]

These people, and many others, have refused to let a hearing handicap bully them. Abraham Lincoln once said, "Most men are about as happy as they make up their minds to be." We could add that most hearing-impaired people are about as handicapped as they allow themselves to be.

What does the future hold? The U.S. Department of Health, Education, and Welfare makes the following encouraging statement in a pamphlet entitled *Hearing Loss:* "Because of the flow of research progress in hearing disorders—the progress in prevention, in earlier diagnosis, and in improved treatment—the present is a fortunate time for the hard-of-hearing person to live in, and the future looks increasingly bright."[14]

That future is your future. You have a challenge to face. Are you going to take what you have left and stay in the contest? It's up to you.

2

How does the hearing mechanism work?

When my car quits on me, I am totally helpless. I don't know a spark plug from a piston, and I couldn't trace the path of the gasoline from the fuel tank through the engine to the exhaust pipe if my life depended on it. To understand what's wrong with the car engine, you need to know how the parts work together when the car is running *normally.*

In the same way, if you have a hearing loss, you need a definite concept of the structure and function of the various parts of the ear so that you can understand the causes, treatment, and rehabilitation procedures that relate to your particular problem. First, to get a clear idea of how the human ear reacts to auditory stimuli, we need to know a little bit about the physical nature of sound.

What is a sound wave? All sound originates with a vibration of some sort. Voice sounds, for instance, occur when air is forced through the vocal folds, causing them to vibrate. These vibrations cause the surrounding molecules of air to bump into one another, setting sound waves into motion. A sound wave, then, is merely a pattern of movement of air molecules, extending outward from a point of vibration.

Here's an analogy to help you visualize how a sound wave travels through the air from its source to reach your ear. Have you ever seen a group of restless children waiting in line in front of a movie theater? What happens when the boy at the end of the line gives the cute little girl in front of him a big shove? She bumps into the child ahead of her, he bumps the next one, and so on until the forward movement travels all the way through the line. The poor little tyke at the head of the line ends up getting banged against the door. By this time, the cute little girl who got the first shove has caught her balance and reacts by moving backward. Each child in turn then pulls back until the little fellow in front is no longer squeezed against the door. Now suppose that the big boy in back continues to shove at regular intervals. The movement would keep going back and forth through the line, and the tot in the front would bump into the door in a repeating pattern. Now think of the boy who is doing the shoving as the vibrator, or sound source, and all the children in the line as air particles that are being set into motion by the vibrator. The theater door would be comparable to the eardrum that is receiving the vibrations of the sound wave. Notice in this analogy that the boy in the back of the line who is doing the shoving doesn't move to the front of the line. In the same way, the movement of each air molecule is purely local. It moves forward, then backward, and finally comes to rest in its original position.[1] My little boy has a toy called a Slinky, which is a long, loosely coiled spring. If you've ever seen one of these toys in operation, you can get a pretty good idea of how sound waves move. Each coil merely moves back and forth, but you can see the "wave" travel all the way from one end of the spring to the other and back again.

These illustrations are fine as far as they go, but we need to extend them a little bit to get a true picture of the movement of sound waves. Sound waves don't just move straight ahead in one direction. They are three-dimensional in that they radiate out in all directions from the sound source, even though the impulse may be stronger in one direction (in front of the speaker, for instance) than in others.

With this picture in mind, we are ready to talk about two characteristics of sound that are important to your understanding of the type and degree of *your* hearing loss. These qualities are *frequency* and *intensity.*

What makes some sounds high pitched and others low pitched? The frequency of a sound wave depends on how fast or slow the vibrations are. The speed of vibration is measured in cycles per second. For instance, in the illustration above, one complete cycle occurs when the "shove" goes all the way through the line of children and back again to the boy who started it. If that boy kept shoving at, say, five shoves a second, the frequency of the wave would be five cycles per second. In sound waves, the more cycles that occur in a second, the higher the frequency, or pitch, of the tone. Until the last few years, frequency was noted as *cycles per second* (cps). By international agreement, frequency units are now designated as *hertz* (abbreviated Hz.) in honor of the German scientist who pioneered studies of sound waves. So when you have a hearing test, you'll know that the term hertz (or Hz) on your audiogram refers to frequency. To give you some idea of how cps, or hertz, relates to pitch, middle C on the piano is 261.6 Hz. This means that, when you strike the middle C key, the surrounding air molecules are displaced 261.6 times in a second. *Frequency,* then, refers to an event happening in the physical world. *Pitch,* on the other hand, refers to the psychological sensation that goes with that event.

Can the human ear hear all frequencies? No. There are many sounds that are outside the range of the human ear. As you probably know, if you have a dog, you can call him with a whistle that is pitched much too high for you to hear. Not all people have the same range of audible frequencies, but generally speaking, about the lowest frequency an adult with normal hearing can perceive is 20 Hz and the highest is around 20,000 Hz. It's always fascinated me to think that there's a whole symphony of sound going on around us that we can't hear at all. It's probably a good thing, though. If wc could hear all sounds, it might be like setting up permanent residence in Grand Central Station. The normal ear hears some frequencies better than others. The ear is most sensitive to the frequencies from 1,000 Hz to 4,000 Hz. It can hear much softer sounds in these frequencies than in frequencies above or below the range of 1,000–4,000 Hz. Most audiometers (electronic hearing-testing machines) are equipped to test the frequencies of 125, 250, 500, 750, 1,000, 1,500, 2,000, 3,000, 4,000, 6,000, and 8,000 Hz. The frequencies that are most essential to the understanding of speech are those in the range between 500 Hz and 4,000 Hz. This is an important fact for you to know, and we'll come back to it in Chapter 6 when we talk about what the results of your hearing tests mean.

Of course, most of the sounds we hear are made up of a combination of tones of different frequencies. Single-frequency sounds are called pure tones, and these are the sounds you hear when your hearing is being tested with an audiometer. Pure tones do not occur often in nature, but they are useful in testing to determine the *pattern* of your hearing loss, which is important for diagnosis and hearing aid adjustment.

Besides frequency, there is one other physical property of sound you need to be on speaking terms with. I'm referring to intensity, or loudness.

What causes variations in the loudness of sound? Remember our line of children outside the movie theater? If the boy who was doing the shoving gave the girl in front of him just a gentle nudge, the movement would still pass through the line, but the child in front would barely tap the door. On the other hand, if the shover was a bully, he might crash into her with such force that the boy in front would smash into the door, almost breaking the glass. Have you ever said, "Stop that noise! It's breaking my eardrums!"? That's because the displaced air particles are striking your eardrum with such force that it's actually painful. *Intensity* refers to the actual strength of the vibration, while *loudness* refers to the listener's reaction to it, so a signal of a given *intensity* may sound *louder* to a person with normal hearing than it does to you.

How is loudness, or intensity, measured? Intensity is usually measured with an instrument called a *sound-level meter.* The results are expressed in *decibels.* In a hearing test given with an audiometer, a zero-decibel level of loudness is the level at which the "normal" human ear can just barely hear a particular sound. Usually, if you can hear a tone at a level of up to 15 or 20 decibels of loudness, your hearing for that frequency is considered to be within normal limits. Sound generally becomes painful to the normal ear at about 135 to 140 decibels of intensity, as measured by a sound-level meter. Normal conversation averages about 60 decibels, in sound pressure level.

Now that we know something about how sound waves operate and have some understanding of frequency and intensity, let's look at the various parts of the hearing mechanism to see how these sound waves are transmitted to the brain.

The ear is one of the most complex structures in the human body. Even before a baby is born, the ear is the first organ of special sense to become differentiated. In fact, responses to sound can be demonstrated in a fetus of twenty six weeks.[2]

The ear is housed within the temporal bone, the hardest bone of the body, to provide adequate protection to its delicate parts. Please refer to Figure 2.1 to locate the various parts of the ear as we discuss each one.

The human ear consists of three main parts: the outer ear, the middle ear, and the inner ear.

What is the function of the outer ear? When you think of the ear, you usually think of the only part you can see—that shell-shaped projection on the side of the head, which is a flap of skin-covered cartilage. Actually, this part of your hearing mechanism contributes very little to your ability to hear, unless of course you happen to be a dog, a rabbit, or one of the other four-footed creatures that can move its

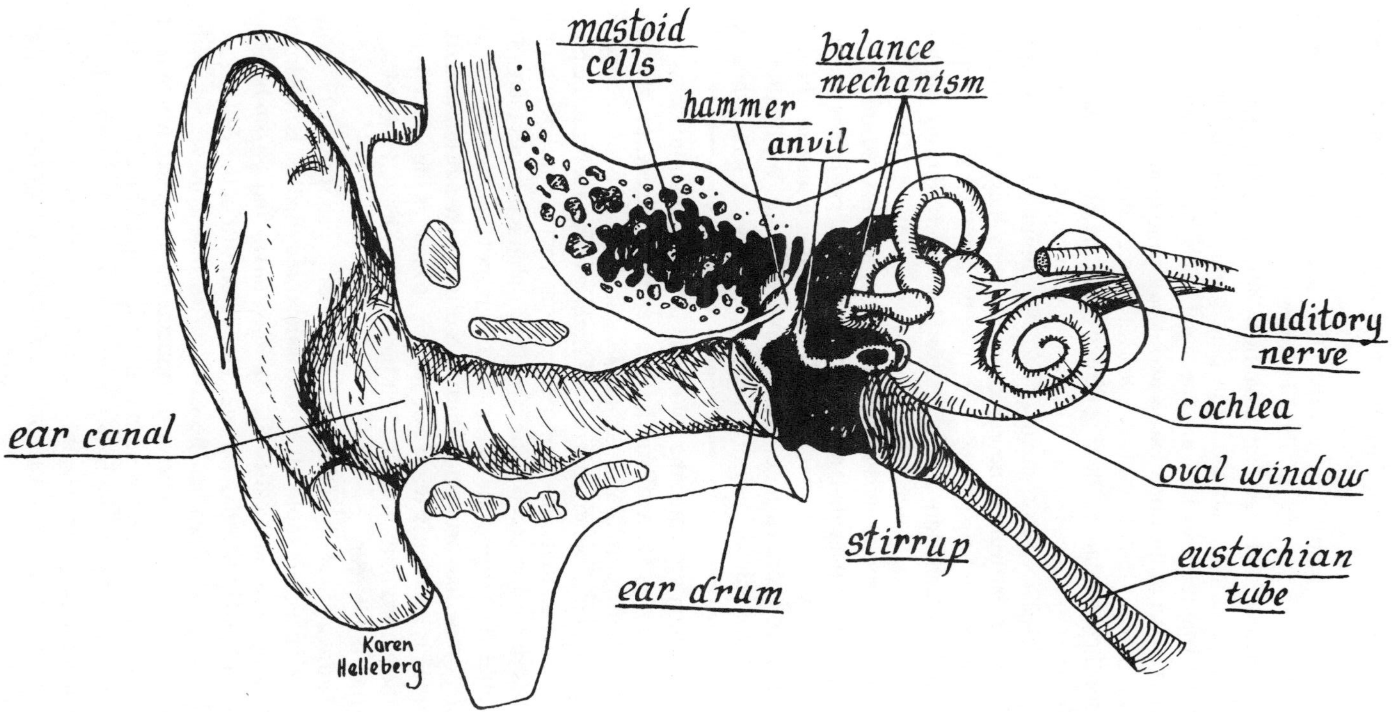

Figure 2.1. The human ear

external ears to help locate the direction sounds are coming from. We've all seen dogs perk up their ears when they hear a faint sound, and it's possible that man may have been able to use his ears in this way at one time. Now, about all this part of our ear can do for us is to direct the sound waves into the ear canal. This canal, which is also considered part of the outer ear, is about 1/4 inch in diameter and a little more than an inch long, and it leads to the eardrum. You usually can't see the eardrum by looking directly into the ear because there's a slight bend in the ear canal. That's why your physician or otologist uses a funnel-shaped instrument called a speculum when he wants to examine your eardrum. The ear canal contains hairs and wax-producing glands that help to keep dust, insects, and other small particles away from the eardrum. Ear wax also has bacteria-killing qualities that guard against infection from microorganisms. Often, these glands get overambitious and secrete too much wax, so that a wax plug is created in the canal, and causes a hearing loss. This is one reason why it's very important to see your doctor if you suspect a hearing problem, before you rush out and buy a hearing aid. We'll talk more about this problem in Chapter 3 when we discuss conductive hearing losses. The inner end of the ear canal is completely closed off by the eardrum, which separates the outer ear from the middle ear.

What, exactly, is the eardrum? It's a semitransparent, pearly gray membrane that is circular in shape; its diameter is about the size of the eraser end of a pencil. It's dented slightly inward toward the middle ear cavity so that, as a loudspeaker constructed similarly, it provides less distortion and broader frequency characteristics than a flat disc would. The sound waves (displaced air molecules) strike against this membrane like drumsticks hitting a drum. Like a drumhead, this membrane is kept fairly tense by a muscle, so that as the sound waves strike the eardrum, it picks up their pattern of vibration and passes it on to the middle ear.

What happens in the middle ear? The middle ear is a cavity about the size of an aspirin tablet. It contains the three smallest bones in the human body, popularly called the *hammer, anvil,* and *stirrup* because they resemble a blacksmith's forge. The outermost of these bones, the hammer, is pressed against the eardrum so that it moves when the eardrum vibrates. The hammer is connected to the anvil, which is, in turn, connected to the stirrup, so that something like a chain reaction occurs as these three little bones move together in tune with the vibrations of the eardrum. The innermost bone in the chain, the stirrup, has a footplate that presses against the membrane covering the opening to the inner ear, called the *oval window.* You can see how these three tiny bones act as a bridge across the cavity of the middle ear, transmitting the sound wave vibrations from the eardrum to the inner ear.

What causes my ears to "pop" when I'm driving in the mountains or flying in an airplane? There's a "ventilator," called the eustachian tube, that connects the middle ear with the nasopharynx (the part of the throat just back of the nasal passages). Normally this tube, which is approximately 1½ inches long, is collapsed; so the opening is closed off. But when changes in outside air pressure occur, the tube opens up to let air in or out. If it weren't for the action of this tube, the eardrum would be forced painfully outward and inward as air pressure increased or decreased with altitude changes. Sometimes, the eustachian tube needs a little help from you; so you swallow, chew gum, or yawn to open it up. When you have a bad cold, the eustachian tube gets plugged up; so it's not a good idca to fly when you have a head cold.

What happens in the inner ear? When the stirrup bone of the middle ear vibrates against the oval window, the sound waves pass into the inner ear, which contains a little snail-shaped mechanism called the *cochlea.* About the size of a pea, the cochlea is the hearing part of the inner ear. It is filled with fluid and contains the Organ of Corti, which is the sensory end organ of hearing. Inside the Organ of Corti are thousands of tiny hair cells that respond to the vibrations the sound waves make in the fluid. The hair cells pass the sensations on to nerve fibers in the auditory nerve. This nerve carries the signals to the brain where, finally, this intricate game of pass-it-on is complete, and you experience the miracle of hearing, attaching a meaning to the sensation of sound.

If this whole process seems very complex, maybe we can simplify it with another analogy, because it's important for you to be able to visualize the entire sequence in order to fully understand your own particular hearing problem. Imagine a group of twelve people standing in a line holding hands. The first person in the line (the sender, or speaker) and the last one (the receiver, or listener) have worked out a code for transmitting messages (speech). Let's say, for example, that one hand squeeze represents the message, "Help me." The sender squeezes the hand of the person next to him, an action comparable to setting the air molecules into vibration. The second person squeezes the hand of the third person, which represents the sound waves being gathered in by the external ear; that person squeezes hand number

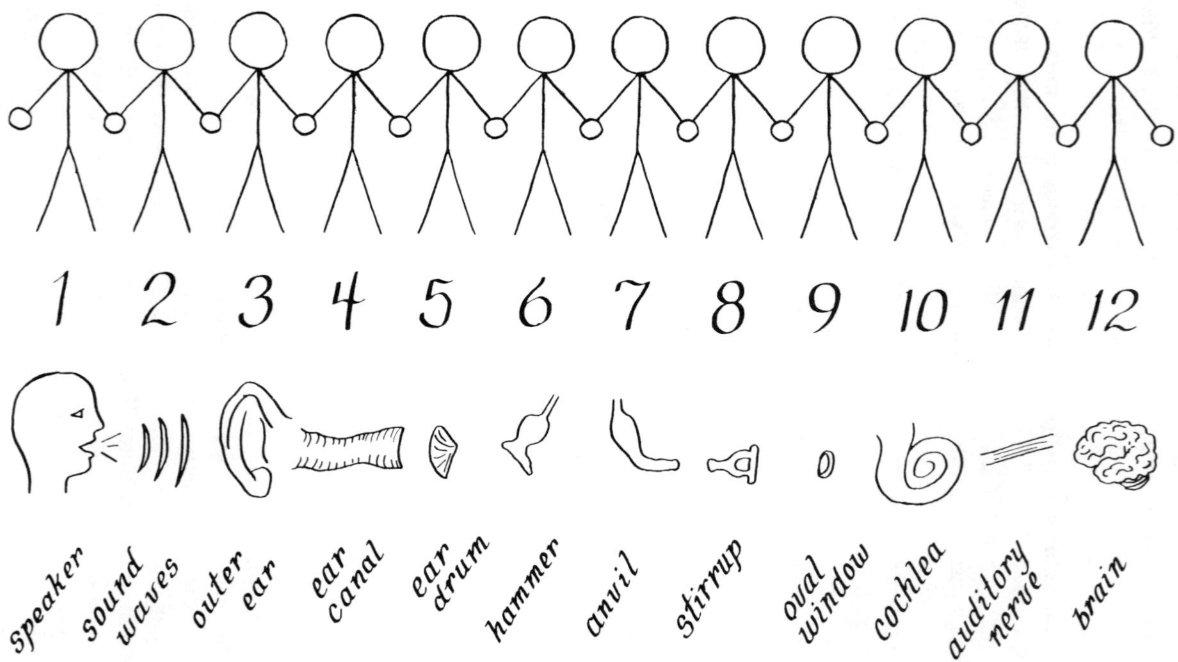

Figure 2.2. How sound signals travel from their source to the brain.

four, passing the message into the ear canal; number four squeezes the hand of the fifth person, who represents the eardrum; hands six, seven, and eight (the middle ear bones) pass on number five's squeeze to person number nine (the oval window). When the tenth person's hand is squeezed, the message has reached the cochlea and the hair cells of the Organ of Corti. All that remains is for number ten to squeeze the hand representing the auditory nerve, and the twelfth person in the line, who represents the brain, decodes the message and says aloud, "Number one needs help." Now study Figure 2.2 to get a clear picture of the whole sequence. I don't know about you, but just thinking about the intricacy and complexity of this perfectly designed mechanism fills me with a deep sense of awe and reverence.

Sometimes, though, even a masterpiece includes flaws. You can see from Figure 2.2 that the message does not get through until all twelve hands have been squeezed. So, if one of the hands along the way should become paralyzed, or numb, or weak, then the signal may continue on, but number twelve will have trouble decoding the feeble or distorted cue. Similarly, *no hearing takes place* until the sound waves have passed all the way from their source through the air, the outer, middle, and inner ear and into the brain. Let this illustration bake in your mental oven for a while, and we'll come back to it when we discuss your own hearing problem in Chapters 3 and 4.

What is the purpose of this involved chain of events? All of this passing on of sound waves from one ear structure to another does seem uncalled-for, but each step is necessary. In water animals, such as fish, auditory signals can be transmitted directly from the water in which they live to the fluid of the inner ear. But since man exists in an *air-filled* environment and the Organ of Corti rests within a fluid medium in the inner ear, a mechanism is needed to adapt the energy of sound from an air medium to a fluid medium. The middle ear acts as a converter for this purpose. The action of the middle-ear bones also serves to increase the force of the vibrations that travel from the eardrum to the oval window. In the inner ear, sound energy is converted at the Organ of Corti into electrical energy in order to stimulate the auditory nerve endings. Obviously, without these important changes along the way, the airborne auditory message could not be transmitted.

Is man capable of hearing sounds that are not transmitted through the air? Since the inner ear is enclosed in the temporal bone, direct vibration of this bone causes movement of the inner-ear fluid. If your head is pressed against a solid surface, such as the floor, vibrations can pass through that surface directly into your skull, and you hear sounds by bone conduction. By pressing your head against a railroad track, you can hear a train coming long before you could hear the sound of its engine by air conduction. We also hear our own voices through bone conduction. This happens because the vibrations of our vocal folds are transmitted directly to the bones of our skull. Of course, if we have a normal outer and middle ear, we also hear our own voices through air conduction at the same time. Have you ever listened to your voice on a tape recorder? If so, it probably sounded strange to you. This is because you are used to hearing your voice by a combination of air and bone conduction. When you hear it on tape, you are hearing it only by air conduction, which is the way others hear you.

Hearing tests should *always* be given both by air conduction (through headphones) and by bone conduction (through a vibrator placed on the mastoid bone just behind the ear), unless the air conduction test proves that your hearing is normal. This is extremely important because, if there is a significant difference between what you can hear by air conduction and what you can hear by bone conduction, this would indicate you have a conductive type of loss, which may be correctable without the use of a hearing aid. We'll talk some more about air conduction and bone conduction testing in Chapter 6.

Does the inner ear have any function besides hearing? Yes. The inner ear is more than an end organ for hearing; it also contains the organ that makes it possible for you to keep your balance. Joining the cochlea are three semicircular canals, which also contain fluid and hair cells. As your head changes position, the fluid in these canals moves around, stimulating the hair cells in different parts of the organ, which in turn send messages to the brain that help you maintain your balance. This is why dizziness often accompanies inner ear infections.

Why do we need two ears? Hearing serves an important purpose in addition to the reception of sound. It provides for spatial orientation. If both of your ears are normal, or both are equally defective, you can close your eyes and still know where I'm standing as I speak to you from various parts of the room. If you're walking along a road, you can tell which direction a car is coming from before it comes into sight. If you're at a party, you can follow the conversation easily as it shifts from one person to another around the room. Sounds are fuller and richer and have more depth for you if both ears are normal. That's why so many people invest in stereophonic record players, which direct the sound to the listener from more than one direction. This ability to localize sound is called *binaural* (two-ear) hearing.

How does binaural hearing provide this spatial orientation? When sound waves come from a single source, they reach the ear closer to the sound a fraction of a second before they reach the other ear. By some amazing process in the brain, we are able to detect this infinitesimal time difference and attach a place meaning to it. Even very young babies turn their heads toward the direction from which their mother's voice is coming. The phenomenon of binaural hearing is an important concept for you to grasp if you have a hearing problem. It may affect your decision about corrective measures, and we'll come back to it when we discuss hearing aid selection in Chapter 7 and suggestions to your family and friends in Chapter 15.

What things interfere with normal hearing? Obviously, even a person whose hearing mechanism is not defective sometimes has trouble hearing. Sounds may be distorted when they reach the ear, by such physical interferences as walls and doors. If you're in the bedroom, you may hear your daughter and her boyfriend talking in the living room, but, strain as you will, you may not be able to make out what they're saying (much to their relief, no doubt!). This is because the wall blocks out certain frequencies and lets others pass through; so the pattern of what you hear is not the same as the original sound pattern. This is also what happens in certain types of hearing loss. The hard-of-hearing person hears the *voices,* if his hearing for the lower frequencies is normal, but he may not be able to *understand* what is being said because his high-frequency hearing loss cuts out most of the consonant sounds.

Another thing that affects normal hearing occurs when the sound traveling to the ear meets another sound along the way, such as a noise or another voice. The second sound messes up the pattern of the original sound waves; so the message is garbled by the time your ear picks it up. You can see that, if you have a hearing loss that makes speech understanding difficult to begin with, intervening sounds can disconnect that communication line completely. That's why you get so edgy when you're trying to watch TV or carry on a conversation and your little boy is going "vroom, vroom" with his toy car in the middle of the living room floor. Say! Show this paragraph to your normal-hearing wife, or husband, or children. They need to know what you're up against!

For lower forms of life, hearing is mostly a defense mechanism; but for the human being, it's much more. Because communication is so important to man, hearing is closely tied up with his feeling of belonging and his sense of well-being. Not only do our ears provide us with warning signals of all kinds, but through them we can react to the warmth of a compliment, the pain of an insult, or the aesthetic pleasure of a song or symphony.

If you have a hearing loss, you want to know what has caused it and what can be done to correct it or to compensate for it. If your telephone is out of order, you need to know, first of all, what is causing the problem. Is the outdoor line down? Is there some part of the receiver that is not making an adequate contact? Do you need an attachment that will amplify the signal? Can the problem be corrected by cleaning out an obstruction in the mechanism or replacing a defective part? Let's assume that, after all these things have been checked out, the experts from the phone company tell you that you're going to have to get along with a weak or distorted auditory reception. Are you going to quit using the phone and adopt a bitter and defeated attitude? You could do that, OR you *could* get busy with the task of finding other ways to supplement the input from your defective equipment.

In the following chapters, we'll try to answer your questions about *why* you have a hearing problem, *what* can be done to correct it and/or to keep it from getting worse, and finally, *how* you can compensate for what cannot be corrected. Please know that, even if your hearing loss is not medically correctable, there are countless ways in which you can improve your ability to communicate and rise above your handicap to attain a full measure of life. So let's get going.

3

Do I have a conductive hearing loss?

Veronica and Jeff both have severe hearing losses, but when they met at a local "deaf club" dinner and started comparing notes, they found that, though they may have had *other* things in common, their hearing losses were about as different as birds and fish are. Veronica's voice was almost a whisper, while Jeff spoke in loud, harsh tones. Veronica could hear speech quite well if people shouted loudly enough, but one of Jeff's pet peeves was people who shout. Jeff couldn't stand noise, but Veronica heard her best in noisy places. He could hear people talking, but he couldn't understand what they said. They both had trouble with head noises, but Veronica described hers as a buzzing sound, while Jeff's ears seemed to be constantly ringing. Veronica's hearing loss had been caused by repeated ear infections, but Jeff had never had an earache in his life. He had worked for years in a machine shop though, and his father and sister were also hard-of-hearing.

Obviously, hearing losses differ not only in *degree* but also in type, causes, and symptoms. It is essential for you to have a clear understanding of these differences so that you will know what you can expect in the way of treatment, possible corrective measures, hearing and speech conservation, and rehabilitation procedures.

This chapter on the symptoms and causes of conductive impairment and the next one, which concerns sensori-neural and central hearing problems, are in *no way* intended to encourage self-diagnosis! Only your physician or otologist can diagnose your particular hearing problem, and you should *always* seek professional help at the first sign of hearing loss. These chapters may help you, though, to better understand and accept their diagnoses and recommendations. With this in mind, we'll try to answer some of your questions about *conductive* hearing impairments.

How many types of hearing defects are there? Basically, there are three major types of hearing losses: (1) poor conduction of sound to the sense organ (conductive loss), (2) abnormality of the sense organ or its nerve (sensori-neural loss), and (3) impairments that result from a flaw in the central nervous system. In some hard-of-hearing persons, more than one of these factors is involved. When this is the case, we use the term *mixed impairment.*

What is a conductive hearing loss? You will remember that, in Chapter 2, we said the hearing mechanism is divided into three parts: the outer, middle, and inner ear. If the inner ear and nerve pathways are normal but something is wrong in the outer or middle ear, then the impairment is *conductive.* In other words, if the sound could just get through to the inner ear, it could be heard clearly. Have you ever received a long-distance telephone call in which you could barely hear the caller because of a poor connection, even though your phone itself was in good working condition? This situation is similar to that of a conductive hearing loss. The parts of the body that perceive and interpret sound (the sense organ of the inner ear and the brain) are ready and waiting, but there's a defective connection somewhere in the outer or middle ear that weakens the sound signal before it can get through to the inner ear.

What are some of the symptoms of conductive hearing loss? If you have a conductive hearing loss, you are probably inclined to speak with a relatively *quiet voice.* This is because we normally regulate the loudness of our voices by the way we ourselves hear them. When we speak, part of the sound of our own voice is transmitted directly through our head bone into our inner ear. Since the person with the conductive loss has a normal inner ear, his own voice sounds louder to him than the voices of others, which have to go through his defective outer and middle ear before he can hear them. So he naturally softens his own voice to match the way other people's voices sound to him.

Another symptom of conductive loss is the *ability to hear speech well in noisy surroundings.* In fact, if you have this type of loss you can usually hear speech *better* in the presence of noise than you can in a quiet place! This is because people with normal hearing speak softly in a quiet room but raise their voices in a noisy place, such as a dance hall or a busy restaurant. Because your conductive loss cush-

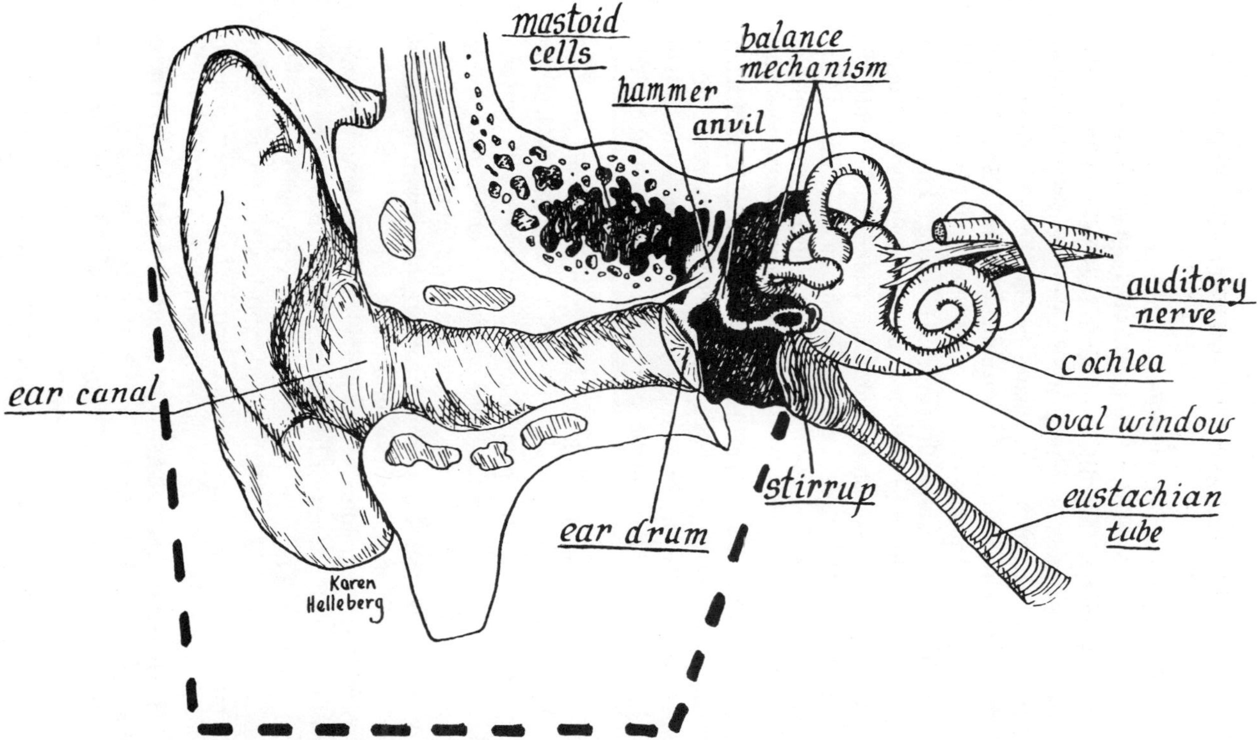

Figure 3.1. Conductive hearing losses are those in which the defect is in the outer or middle ear, as marked by the broken line in the above diagram.

ions you against the background noise, you benefit from the increased loudness with which those around you are speaking. In fact, you may even hear better in such situations than your normally hearing friends do, because your hearing loss has trained you to lipread. It has also been suggested that "the continuous presence of noise in the background, as in a moving vehicle or a factory, 'sensitizes' the conducting mechanism in such a way that it becomes more receptive to the sounds of speech within that environment."[1] This ability to hear better in noisy surroundings than in quiet ones was first noted by Thomas Willis in the seventeenth century. He wrote, "I heard from a credible person, that he once knew a woman, though she were deaf, yet so long as a drum was beating within her chamber, she heard every word perfectly. Therefore, her husband kept a drummer on purpose for his servant, that by that means he might have some converse with his wife!"[2]

Another characteristic that distinguishes conductive loss from sensori-neural loss is the fact that a patient with a conductive problem *understands* well what he hears as long as speech is made loud enough for him. As we'll see in the next chapter, this is not true of the individual with a sensori-neural loss.

Furthermore, if your loss is conductive, you can *tolerate loud sounds* that would cause discomfort to a person with normal hearing and that would be actually painful to many persons with sensori-neural losses. The reason is that your conductive impairment serves as a protector to your inner ear in the same way that wearing ear plugs does for a person with normal hearing. Here again, this is not true for a person with a sensori-neural loss.

A person with a conductive loss is likely to have about the same degree of loss for all pitches, or frequencies. With this type of hearing problem, if you can't hear the phone ringing, you probably can't hear a foghorn blowing, either. High sounds and low sounds are about equally impaired for you, and this is called a *"flat" pattern* of loss. We'll go into patterns of loss in more detail in Chapter 6.

Are you bothered by continuous or intermittent head noises? These annoying sounds may be in one ear or both ears or may seem to be just unlocalized in the head. The otologist and audiologist call these head noises *tinnitus.* Tinnitus is one of the most bothersome symptoms of impaired hearing, often causing nervousness and sometimes sleeplessness. It seems to get worse when you're tired or under emotional strain. Still, it may relieve your mind a little to know that it does *not* mean that your hearing is getting worse, nor will it actually "drive you crazy," though you probably use that expression to describe how annoying it is.

What causes tinnitus in people with conductive impairments? A piece of ear wax or other foreign matter pressing against the ear canal can cause it. Some medicines, such as quinine and aspirin, can cause it in people who are especially sensitive to them, and alcoholic beverages can increase these noises. Usually, the sound is described as a humming, buzzing, or ringing noise. Another kind of tinnitus is a gurgling noise, which is caused by liquid in the middle ear, usually following an upper respiratory or ear infection or an allergic reaction.

Very often, when conductive impairments are corrected medically or surgically, the nuisance of tinnitus disappears. If correction is not possible, your doctor *may* prescribe a sedative, but continued use is not advisable. Norton Canfield, M.D., points out that "pre-occupation with some absorbing interest or hobby is the best antidote for noisy ears." He also suggests background music and offers hope that "research now in progress will result in more important data on this perplexing problem."[3]

Is conductive hearing loss likely to result in total deafness? Not if it's a purely conductive loss. If the sense organ of the inner ear is normal and the impairment is only in the outer or middle ear, the loss cannot be greater than about sixty decibels. This is because, once that level of loudness is reached, bone conduction takes over, transmitting the sound to the normal inner ear. So the person with the purely conductive loss can always hear very loud speech, and he finds it easy to adjust to a hearing aid.

What are the causes of conductive hearing impairment? Let's begin with the outer ear. By far the most common cause of outer ear malfunction is a wax plug in the ear canal. In most people, the ear wax secretion is soft and works its way out of the ear, where it is removed by washing. In some people, though, the wax is much harder and tends to collect gradually until it finally closes off the canal completely. Usually, no hearing loss is noticed until the blockage is complete; so it's rather common for a person with this problem to complain of a sudden, dramatic loss of hearing. Sometimes this occurs after swimming, because ear wax absorbs water, and so wax that has been collecting for months or years may swell up enough to complete the closure. Don't be embarrassed about this problem. It has nothing to do with personal cleanliness. You could wash your ears every day and still develop a wax plug if your wax-secreting glands are overactive or if the secretion is abnormally hard. In fact, excessive cleaning of the ears may even aggravate the problem by pushing the wax in further or preventing it from working its way out naturally. A wax plug should always be removed by a physician or otologist. The skin of the ear canal is delicate and very easily scratched, and scratches can lead to infection. In addition, damage to the eardrum can result from probing in the ear canal with a bobby pin, pencil, or toothpick. Wax removal is a simple procedure for your doctor. Don't take a chance on creating a more serious problem by poking around in your ear. In Chapter 5, we'll discuss the ways in which the doctor may remove a wax plug.

Once a wax plug has been removed, is the problem apt to recur? Yes. It may do so again after only a few weeks or months, or maybe even years later. It is sometimes necessary to establish a schedule for periodic removal of wax by the otologist.

Are there other things besides wax that may block the canal? Children sometimes stuff such objects as corn kernels or peanuts into the ear and forget about them until they begin to experience pain or hearing loss. A more common problem in adults is a swelling of the canal walls caused by such skin conditions as eczema or dermatitis. The itching that accompanies these irritations may cause the person to scratch his ear, thereby introducing infection and further swelling. Always consult your physician if you have a problem with itchy ears.

Individuals who do a lot of swimming may develop bony growths in the ear canal, which make the passages narrower. These obstructions may result in skin diseases or excessive wax accumulation, either of which may close the canal and result in hearing loss.

In addition to these outer-ear problems, there are various middle-ear conditions that trigger hearing impairment.

Can the common earache cause hearing loss? Yes. In fact, earache is the symptom of the most frequent cause of conductive impairment, an infection of the middle ear called *otitis media.* As we explained in Chapter 2, the eustachian tube connects the middle ear with the area at the back of the throat behind the nasal passages. When you have a bad head cold, an allergic condition, an upper respiratory infection such as measles or mumps, or sinusitis, the infection or inflammation can easily pass through the eustachian tube into the middle ear. This often happens as a result of improper nose blowing, which forces mucus into the middle ear. Never pinch your nostrils together when blowing your nose. Press lightly on one nostril at a time and blow gently. Once the infection has been extended into the middle ear, fluid builds up in there, causing pressure against the inside surface of the eardrum. Not only is this painful, but it also causes at least a temporary loss of hearing acuity because the drum and middle-ear bones cannot vibrate freely.

But won't the hearing loss disappear as soon as the infection is cleared up? It may, but prompt medical attention is essential because the temporary loss can easily become permanent.

How does this happen? Without early medical treatment, the pressure behind the eardrum can build up rapidly until the drum breaks. If the broken membrane fails to heal properly, permanent hearing impairment is likely to follow.

Otitis media can also become chronic, and the recurring infections may cause adhesions to form on the bones in the middle ear, damaging or even destroying these essential links in the hearing chain. This may result in permanent hearing disability.

Chronic otitis media is dangerous, not only because of its threat to hearing, but also because it may lead to mastoiditis, which can be fatal. *Always* take an earache to the doctor—and don't wait!

Can enlarged adenoids cause hearing loss? Yes, otitis media can also result from enlarged adenoids that block the eustachian tube, causing the eardrum to be pulled inward. This, too, results in hearing loss because it interferes with the ability of the drum to vibrate. Hearing usually returns to normal when the adenoids are removed. But again, this should be done promptly because the hearing defect can become permanent if fluid is allowed to build up in the middle ear and to remain there long enough to damage those tiny bones.

There's a young man in one of my college classes whose enlarged adenoids began to interfere with his hearing when he was in the second grade. When the family doctor advised surgery, the parents refused, because the boy's father had had adenoid trouble when he was a boy, too, but he "outgrew it." When this young man showed no signs of "outgrowing" the problem, his parents finally agreed to surgery—four years later. By that time, the middle ear was so badly damaged that the hearing loss was permanent. I can't be too harsh in my judgment of this boy's parents because I'm sure they thought they were doing the right thing at the time. But at least I can pass on to *you* the lesson they learned too late, so that if your doctor advises adenoid removal for one of your children, you won't put it off.

What is "glue ear"? Since the use of antibiotics has become common in the treatment of simple otitis media, otologists have grown increasingly aware of a problem these drugs help to create. What happens is this: A patient complains of earache which is diagnosed as otitis media. Antibiotics are prescribed, the infection clears up, and the earache disappears. But the fluid, no longer infectious, remains in the middle-ear cavity, making the ear susceptible to repeated attacks of the infection, and causing reduced hearing acuity. The patient is usually unaware of his hearing loss until both ears are affected. By this time, the fluid has become thickened and gluelike and may have caused permanent deterioration of the middle-ear bones.

Does this mean that antibiotics shouldn't be prescribed for ear infections? Not really, because without the use of antibiotics, a simple middle-ear infection can easily turn into mastoiditis, which can be a serious threat to life itself.

What, then, can be done to prevent "glue ear"? First of all, if your doctor prescribes an antibiotic for an ear infection, be sure to follow his directions for taking it. Do not stop using it as soon as the earache is relieved, but continue with the full course of medication the doctor has prescribed. Also, be sure to have your hearing tested audiometrically after every ear infection to make sure that healing is complete. This is of extreme importance because, if fluid remains in the middle ear, you'll probably not otherwise be aware of it. If your hearing is affected, the otologist may recommend removing the fluid surgically to prevent permanent damage.

Can sinus trouble cause hearing loss? Sinusitis is an inflammation of the linings of the air spaces in the bones of the face around the nose. When infectious material irritates the back of the nose, it may cause swelling around the eustachian tube and, as we have seen, such swelling interferes with the normal functioning of the middle ear. Hearing impairment can be the result. Your doctor can determine, with the help of X-rays, whether or not there is a relationship between your sinus trouble and your hearing loss.

If you have sinus trouble, be especially careful about the use of nasal sprays. They can relieve the congestion temporarily, but if you use them excessively, they can aggravate the problem by causing a rebound reaction that increases the swelling and irritation.

What about smoking and hearing impairment? Canfield describes the relationship well:

> Smoking puts an extra burden on the nose and throat, and these structures cannot function normally when repeatedly so insulted. This is especially true of cigarettes, because the smoke from the burning paper contains irritating substances. Much nose and throat discomfort can be elimi-

> nated merely by ceasing to smoke. The reasons for not smoking are infinitely more potent for people with a hearing loss. Abstinence often convinces even the most skeptical.[4]

Could my hearing loss be caused by my nasal allergies? Yes. If you suffer from hay fever or postnasal swelling due to allergies, your hearing impairment may be improved by the use of prescribed antihistamines or a program of allergy treatment. If simple treatment with antihistamines is not adequate, you should see an allergist. If getting rid of your allergies is not incentive enough, surely improved hearing ability should be.

Can a slap on the ear damage the hearing mechanism? Definitely. A sharp blow to the ear can rupture the eardrum. Such injuries usually heal normally, but they *can* cause a permanent hole, or perforation, in the eardrum. Canfield notes that even "a passionate kiss has been known to rupture the eardrum!"[5] Hmmm. . . .

What other injuries can cause damage to the eardrum? As we mentioned earlier, poking any foreign object into the ear is risky business because, besides possibly scratching the ear canal, it can also rupture the eardrum. Blast injuries in combat are common causes of ruptured eardrums, and even powerful fire crackers can cause such wounds.

An accident that fractures the bony ring in the skull to which the eardrum is attached is likely to break the membrane, so bleeding from the ear following a head injury should always be looked into.

Can the middle-ear bones be damaged by accidental injury? Yes. A head injury, such as often occurs in a car accident, can fracture the temporal bone which houses the hearing mechanism, causing the bones of the middle ear to become disconnected or fractured. Obviously, any severe head injury should be followed by a thorough examination by an otologist!

Can bad teeth cause hearing loss? Indirectly, yes, because of the close relationship between the jaw joint and the ear. If you place your finger in front of your ear and open and close your mouth, you can feel how close the jaw joint is to the hearing mechanism. If your upper and lower teeth don't fit together properly, you may develop swelling and pain around your ear, which can cause loss of hearing. This incorrect meshing of the jaws may be caused by missing teeth, impacted molars, badly decayed teeth, or teeth that have come in crooked. Canfield notes that "in skillful hands some ear symptoms including deafness have been relieved by proper attention to the teeth and jaws."[6]

What is otosclerosis? This is a disease that changes the normally hard bone near the oval window into a soft, spongy bone. As you will remember from our discussion of the hearing mechanism in Chapter 2, the stirrup bone of the middle ear presses against the membrane that covers the oval window, which leads into the inner ear. As the disease of otosclerosis progresses, the stirrup bone may become fixed at this point, so that it cannot move freely enough to transmit sound waves effectively to the inner ear. A conductive hearing impairment results, and the disease may eventually progress to involve the inner ear, causing a sensori-neural complication in addition to the conductive component. Apparently, many people experience the bone changes of otosclerosis without suffering fixation of the stirrup bone and hearing loss. For this reason, even though the disease is itself thought to be hereditary, it may cause hearing loss in a patient with no known family history of defective hearing. It is most prevalent in the white race, and more women than men develop the disease. Hearing loss that is caused by otosclerosis is *usually* first noticed in the late teens or early twenties, although it *can* show up earlier or later in rare instances. Often, the hearing loss becomes apparent, or grows more severe, during pregnancy and childbirth.

Does this mean that a woman with otosclerosis should not have children? Dr. Hallowell Davis would not advise her to avoid pregnancy. In his words, "Otosclerosis may become worse during pregnancy, but since the disease is often progressive during early adulthood in any case, . . . and since pregnancy by no means always accelerates the process, *otosclerosis should not be considered a deterrent to the bearing of children.*"[7]

How severe is the hearing loss caused by otosclerosis? Usually, the hearing impairment progresses (sometimes quite rapidly) from a very mild defect to about forty to fifty decibels of loss and then levels off. Most patients can hear quite well with a hearing aid, but, because inner-ear involvement may develop, the otologist may recommend surgery to correct the condition. (See Chapter 5.)

These, then, are the more common causes of conductive hearing defects, though I want to make it clear that the listing in this chapter is not all-inclusive. Also, because this book is intended primarily for laymen, I have resorted to oversimplification of some highly complex problems. If you want a more detailed, technical description of the processes involved, I refer you to the references that follow.

When, as a child, I complained about foods I disliked, my father always said, "You're lucky to have any food at all. Children are starving in China." Well, I didn't feel lucky, and I resented the comparison. So if you have a conductive loss, I'm not going to tell you that you're lucky. I can tell you, though, that most conductive hearing losses can be improved by medical and/or surgical treatment and that in many cases hearing can be restored completely by these measures. (See Chapter 5.) Even people whose hearing cannot be restored tend to adapt easily to the use of a hearing aid, if their loss is conductive. (See Chapter 8.) In both of these ways, you have a distinct advantage over those who suffer from sensori-neural losses. I'm glad I didn't use the word *lucky.* It doesn't fit. Still, the outlook for you is very encouraging—and, well, there *are* those "children in China". . . .

4

What are the symptoms and causes of sensori-neural hearing losses and central and functional impairments?

"There's something else I should tell you before you test my husband's hearing, Mrs. Helleberg." I sensed a tenseness in the high-pitched voice coming over the phone. "Sometimes I think George really has a hearing loss, and then sometimes I think he is just faking it. You know what I mean?"

"Well, maybe you should tell me what makes you think that, Mrs. B."

"Well for one thing, he never hears the phone or doorbell ringing, or the baby crying, so I'm the one who always has to stop whatever I'm doing and go and take care of things. But the other day I decided to run to the store while he was taking a nap, and almost the minute I started the car, he was at the front door wanting to know where I was going. Now if he *really* had a hearing loss, the sound of the car starting surely wouldn't wake him up—especially since the garage is on the opposite side of the house from the bedroom. Then, too, he often says he can't understand what I'm saying, but just let his best buddy drop by, and he hears every word he says! Does *that* sound like somebody who is hard of hearing?"

"I can answer that better after we've tested his hearing, Mrs. B. There's a chance that he's faking, as you say. There's also a chance that his hearing loss may be very real, in spite of these inconsistencies."

I'll tell you about the results of George's hearing test later in the chapter, but first here's another case I want to share with you.

Susan, a high school senior, was brought home from school one afternoon by the school nurse. Frightened and in tears, she kept holding her ears and saying, "I can't hear anything!" The nurse explained to Susan's mother what had happened. The girl had been hit on the ear by a volleyball, and, when the phys. ed. teacher asked her if she could hear all right, she suddenly realized that she was deaf. Susan was examined thoroughly by several medical specialists, including an otologist and a neurologist, but they found nothing wrong. Still, she couldn't hear, and, as it turned out, there *was* something wrong.

One more case. Twenty-year-old Brian suffered a fractured skull in a car accident that killed his parents. Following the accident, he showed all the signs of deafness, but the results of his pure-tone audiometric tests were normal.

One of the above patients has a *sensori-neural* (sometimes spelled sensorineural or sensory-neural) hearing loss; one of them has what is called *central deafness;* and one of them has a *functional* hearing loss. In this chapter, we'll talk about these three types of hearing impairment.

Let's begin with sensori-neural hearing loss because most people who are born with impaired hearing have this type of problem. It can also descend on you suddenly or creep up on you at any time in your life, particularly as those birthdays begin to add up. You've probably heard it called nerve loss or perceptive deafness.

A sensori-neural hearing loss occurs when the outer- and middle-ear parts are functioning normally but there's something wrong in the inner ear or the nerve pathway to the brain. In Chapter 3, we compared a conductive impairment to a long-distance telephone call with a poor connection that made it difficult for you to hear the caller, even though your phone was in good order. A sensori-neural impairment is just the opposite. All the wires coming into the house are O K, but the phone inside the house (the inner ear or nerve) is out of order. As I explained in Chapter 2, the inner ear is a bony container filled with fluid. This fluid is set into waving motion by the final bone in the middle ear. The different sized sound waves activate various sound-sensitive hair cells in the cochlea. If these hair cells become insensitive, hearing loss results. The Eighth Nerve, or auditory nerve, is the connecting link between the inner ear and the brain. A defect in this nerve also causes loss of hearing acuity.

What are some of the symptoms of sensori-neural hearing loss? If you have this type of impairment, you may *speak in a louder than normal voice.* People may tell you to "stop shouting," or to "hold your voice down a little."

Why the loud voice? As we noted in the last chapter, we normally hear our own voices both by air conduction (from the outside) and by bone conduction (directly through our own head bone). If you have an inner ear or nerve problem, your hearing by bone conduction is not normal, so your own voice doesn't sound very loud to you. You speak more loudly to compensate for this. Have you ever listened to a woman talking while she's sitting under the hair dryer? She automatically raises her voice to make up for the fact that her normal voice sounds faint to her. This is what happens in many cases of sensori-neural hearing loss.

What are some other symptoms of sensori-neural loss? If your loss is of this type, you may have *trouble understanding speech,* even though you hear voices quite clearly. This is because most people with sensori-neural loss, though not all of them, hear the low pitches, or frequencies, better than the high ones. In fact, your hearing may even be normal or close to normal for frequencies up to 500 Hz or even 1,000 Hz (one or two octaves above middle C) and then drop off quite suddenly for frequencies above this level. You can hear voices well, because they are pitched below the level of your loss. But many of the consonant sounds of speech are high-pitched and weak in intensity. So your high-frequency hearing loss causes you to miss these sounds. No wonder the words are hard to decipher! For instance, the words *same, fame,* and *came* may all sound alike to you because you don't hear the beginning or final consonant in any of these words. All you really hear is the vowel—the long *a.* Unless you can pick up clues from watching the speaker's mouth, you're likely to misinterpret what he says.

George, whose wife thought he was faking, had a high-frequency sensori-neural hearing loss. That's why he could hear her car starting (a low-pitched sound) but couldn't hear the phone or doorbell ringing or the baby crying. He had trouble understanding his wife's speech because she had a high-pitched voice. Besides, she often talked to him as she went about her daily household routine; so he couldn't see her lips. His buddy, on the other hand, had a low voice and, when he and George were together, they usually conversed face to face. George, without fully realizing it, was picking up most of the consonant sounds in his friend's speech, not by hearing, but by lipreading.

Of course, if you have this type of hearing loss, it doesn't do any good for people to shout at you, because you can hear their voices. You just can't understand their words, because your inner ear mechanism can't pick up high-pitched consonant sounds. There *are* some

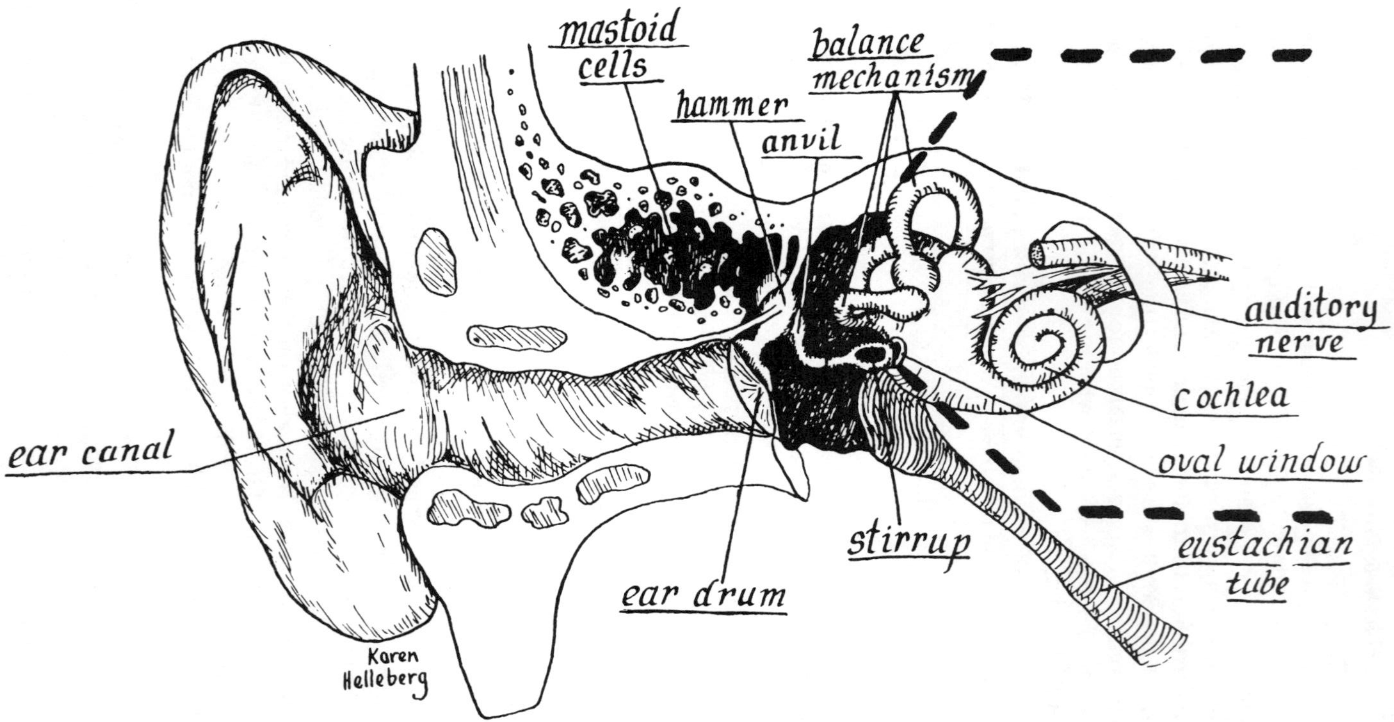

Figure 4.1. As indicated by the broken line in the above diagram, a defect that occurs in the inner ear or nerve pathway to the brain causes a sensori-neural hearing loss.

very specific things you can do to help yourself to better understanding, though. (See Chapters 9 and 10.)

Do you get upset when people shout at you, or do you develop a headache in a noisy place? This may also be a symptom of sensori-neural hearing loss, especially if the defect is in the cochlea of your inner ear. For some reason, this type of impairment causes the *sensation of loudness to build up very rapidly,* even when the actual intensity of the sound increases only moderately. Say, for instance, that you're having your hearing tested with an audiometer. You may be able to just barely hear a certain tone at fifty decibels of loudness. When the examiner increases the intensity to sixty decibels, the tone may sound quite loud to you. If he turns it up to ninety decibels, it may be painfully loud for you, even though you have a hearing loss for that particular tone. This is why loud noises may bother you even more than they bother a person with normal hearing. This rapid increase in the sensation of loudness is called *recruitment.* This recruitment factor, plus your inability to hear consonant sounds, makes it particularly *difficult for you to hear speech in noisy surroundings.* This makes your problem different from that of the person with a conductive loss, who, as we noted in Chapter 3, often hears *better* in noisy places.

You may also have some *pitch distortion* with a sensori-neural loss. Certain tones may sound higher or lower to you than they really are, or one of your ears may hear the tones normally, while the other ear hears the same tones higher or lower or perceives them as noises instead of pure tones.

What about this ringing in my ears? As in conductive impairments, most people with sensori-neural problems are bothered by head noises, or tinnitus. Usually the pitch of tinnitus is higher in sensori-neural impairments than in conductive impairments.

What causes sensori-neural hearing loss? Let's start at the beginning. As I said earlier, most people who are born with hearing losses have sensori-neural impairment. Some of these are hereditary, some are caused by conditions of the mother during pregnancy, and some happen during the birth process.

Is hereditary deafness very common? John Ballantyne estimates that one third of all cases of congenital deafness (that is, people who are born deaf) are hereditary.[1] In addition to these congenital cases, many people who have normal hearing at birth develop hearing loss in later life as a result of an *inherited tendency* toward defective hearing. The disease of otosclerosis, described in Chapter 3, seems to "run in families," as do some types of purely sensori-neural loss. Sometimes deafness forms a part of a syndrome, or group of symptoms, that are hereditary. Inherited sensori-neural hearing impairment may result from many kinds of abnormalities in the genes. The effect on hearing may be immediate (congenital) or delayed (arising later in life). Researchers have found that, when both parents are congenitally deaf for unexplained reasons, their chances of giving birth to a deaf child are very great. Sometimes, however, deaf children are born to parents with normal hearing. In such cases, each parent may have contributed a recessive gene for deafness, or the baby's hearing may have been damaged during pregnancy or childbirth. If your otologist tells you that your hearing loss might be hereditary, you should consult an expert in medical genetics before having children. There are genetic counseling centers in a number of locations throughout the U.S. You may obtain information about them by writing to The American Genetics Association, 1507 M Street N.W., Washington, DC 20005.

What are some of the physical abnormalities associated with hereditary sensori-neural hearing impairment? There may be an incomplete development of the inner ear, or a chromosome abnormality, or the auditory nerve cells may be particularly susceptible to damage.[2]

What conditions during pregnancy can cause sensori-neural hearing loss in the unborn child? If the mother has German measles (rubella) during the first three months of pregnancy, her baby may be born deaf or have some lesser degree of hearing impairment. Now that medical science has developed a vaccine that prevents German measles, the number of cases of congenital hearing impairment from this cause should begin to decrease. *Every* girl should be immunized against this insidious disease early in life, long before she reaches childbearing age!

The fetus may also suffer impaired development of the ear if the mother contracts other virus diseases, such as mumps and influenza, particularly during the first three months of pregnancy. Fortunately, medical laboratories are now conducting full-scale research into this problem of virus infection. Let's hope that some effective preventive measures will soon be developed that will virtually wipe out this cause of congenital hearing loss!

Another threat to normal development of hearing in babies is the Rh blood factor. When the mother has Rh negative type blood and the father has Rh positive, the baby who inherits his father's Rh positive blood may be in danger. Although a blood transfusion shortly after birth may save the baby's life, there may be permanent damage to his hearing, his brain, or some other physical mechanism. Abnormalities from Rh incompatibility are rare in the first child, but the danger increases with each pregnancy. If you and your spouse have this problem, let your doctor advise you on the risks involved in future pregnancies.

It is also possible that certain drugs taken by the mother during the first three months of pregnancy may damage the baby's developing cochlea. Ballantyne observes that "it is in this period, for example, that abortofacients (drugs taken for the purpose of abortion) are sometimes used, and an unsuccessful attempt to terminate a pregnancy may lead to tragic consequences in the unwanted child."[3]

Syphilis that is transmitted from a mother to her baby during pregnancy may also cause the child to develop a hearing loss, either during the first two years of his life or at the time of puberty.

What about birth injuries and hearing? Ballantyne estimates that at least twenty percent of babies who have impaired hearing acquired the defects at the time of birth.[4] Among the causes of these impairments are: toxemias in the mother, prematurity, birth injury, lack of oxygen, or jaundice. In quite a few cases of congenital birth-induced deafness, the cause is, frankly, unknown. Research is lowering the number of these unknown causes, so we can hope for fewer cases of hearing damage for babies of the future.

What are some of the causes of sensori-neural hearing impairments that are acquired at various ages throughout life? Sensori-neural hearing loss can develop at any age from such causes as diseases, injury, tumor, drugs, or interruption of the blood supply to the cochlea. Or it can be brought on by that sly fellow that sneaks up on all of us—advanced age.

What diseases can rob you of your sharp hearing acuity? Some of these thiefs are now preventable by immunization; they include measles, mumps, whooping cough, and diphtheria. Others, such as scarlet fever and meningitis, often respond well to antibiotics. Sometimes flu and other viruses can cause hearing damage. All of the above diseases may also cause conductive hearing loss when middle-ear infection is involved. If the disease produces a toxic effect on nerve endings in the cochlea, sensori-neural loss may result. You should have your hearing tested following any of these infectious diseases, especially measles, mumps, and meningitis. Your test results may be normal, but on the other hand, if there *is* a loss, early detection is vital.

What about sensori-neural loss caused by tumor? Tumors that grow in the area between the cochlea and the auditory nerve cause sensorineural loss by creating pressure on this nerve. Usually only one ear is affected in this way, but, more rarely, both ears can be involved. Often the hearing loss is the first symptom that alerts the doctor to the presence of such a tumor.

What is Meniere's disease? It's an affliction that causes tinnitus, vertigo (dizziness), nausea, pain, and hearing loss. These symptoms often come and go for no obvious reason. Increased pressure in the fluid of the inner ear causes the symptoms, but there is some question about what brings on this increased pressure. Allergy may be involved, and emotional factors may trigger attacks. Norton Canfield asserts that "it seems to occur usually in a specific type of person—those who are intelligent, sensitive, and conscientious but frustrated in their life situation because they are trying to cope with impossible situations. It sometimes hits as the aftermath of intense emotional strain or profound grief."[5] It seems to be more common in women than in men. Recruitment (that rapid increase in the sensation of loudness) is often very severe for the patient suffering from Meniere's disease. The disease usually begins between the ages of 35 and 55, and the hearing loss that comes with it generally affects the low tones before the high tones. Hearing tends to worsen with each attack. Fortunately, Meniere's disease usually occurs primarily in one ear, so the sufferer may be able to hear well enough for purposes of daily life.

What about the patient who suddenly loses almost all of his hearing "overnight"? This happens sometimes, and like Meniere's disease, is almost always accompanied by tinnitus and sometimes by dizziness. Hayes Newby explains that "such sudden losses are thought to be due to an interruption of blood supply to the cochlea, probably a spasm of the cochlear artery. If the condition persists more than a few hours, the cochlea suffers irreparable damage and the hearing loss becomes permanent."[6]

The director of the Veterans Administration's hearing-aid program, Dr. G. Donald Causey, says that any sudden loss of hearing should be treated as a medical emergency. It could be caused by a virus or vascular accident, making it potentially a life-and-death matter. Delay of more than twenty-four hours could allow a possibly temporary hearing impairment to become a permanent loss.

If you should suffer a sudden hearing loss, contact your doctor immediately. Most likely, he'll arrange for you to be seen by an otologist without delay. If you cannot reach your doctor, go directly to the emergency department of the hospital.[7]

Can head injuries cause sensori-neural deafness? As we noted in Chapter 3, a fractured skull may damage the middle ear, causing conductive hearing impairment. A few such fractures also rupture the Organ of Corti in the cochlea and cause sensori-neural loss. This usually involves only one ear, though there may be some additional loss in the opposite ear. Damage to hearing is usually severe and permanent.

A blow on the head that results in a concussion may cause hearing impairment, too, but the loss is less severe than with a fracture and generally only temporary. Hearing acuity is usually regained in a few days or weeks.

What kind of hearing loss is caused by blast injuries? Soldiers in combat often notice hearing impairment following exposure to sudden, intense explosions. Blast injuries have even been caused by firecrackers exploding too close to the ear. Damage may be to the middle ear, the inner ear, or both. The blast may cause bleeding in the inner ear or rupture of the Organ of Corti in the cochlea. If your hearing has been damaged by blast injury, the chances are good that you will recover some (maybe even all) of your hearing, but any loss that stays with you for more than six months is likely to be permanent. Sometimes, however, it goes the other way, and you may seem to recover your hearing, only to find it deteriorating gradually later.

How does noise affect hearing acuity? In the blast injuries we've been discussing, the damage is due mainly to the exertion of extreme and sudden *pressure* on delicate structures. There's also a chronic type of noise-induced hearing loss that develops gradually over a period of time in people who are repeatedly exposed to high levels of noise. This includes people who work in noisy factories, or who are exposed to aircraft engine noise, or who operate loud farm machinery, or even musicians who play in rock-and-roll bands. Our world is becoming steadily noisier in the name of progress. When progress begins to rob us of one of our most valuable God-given senses, it seems to me that the time has come to check the price tag.

People differ in their susceptibility to noise, so it's very important that all applicants for jobs in high-noise areas be screened for such sensitivity before they are employed. Not only is the level of noise important, but the type of noise and the length of exposure is also crucial. For instance, most people show a temporary loss of hearing acuity at the end of an eight-hour working day in a noisy factory or after a day of firing on the rifle range or an evening of playing in a pop band. This is called *temporary threshold shift,* and hearing usually returns to normal after a day or two of noise-free rest. But there comes a time when the score begins to add up. With repeated exposures, the hearing level continues to go up and down. After a while, instead of returning to normal after a period of rest, hearing level returns to almost normal, then to less than normal, then to much less than normal, until the damage has become permanent. The most insidious thing about noise-induced hearing loss is that it very often sneaks in unnoticed. By the time the loss is great enough to make you say, "I don't seem to be hearing as well as I used to," you may have developed a permanent, irreversible hearing loss.

Noise-induced hearing loss typically affects the higher frequencies first. The nerve cells that respond to the frequencies between 3,000 Hz and 6,000 Hz are the most susceptible to noise damage. In fact, an audiogram (hearing test graph) that shows a "dip" at 3,000 Hz, 4,000 Hz, or 6,000 Hz arouses immediate suspicions that the hearing loss is caused by noise exposure. If the person continues to live with noise, the loss will gradually extend to frequencies above and below these areas. A ninety-decibel level of loudness is considered to be unsafe for continued exposure. Through the Occupational Safety and Health Act, the U.S. government is trying to control factory noise levels. In Chapter 11, we'll discuss some specific things you can do to protect the hearing you have left from further invasion by the enemy forces of noise.

What drugs can cause sensori-neural hearing loss? Just as some people are more susceptible to noise-induced hearing loss than others are, some can suffer ear damage from certain drugs that have little effect on others. Even such a common drug as aspirin can cause sensori-neural hearing loss in people whose ears are sensitive to it. Though many people take aspirin regularly without any adverse effect on their hearing, the drug creates a toxic reaction in the inner ear of some people. Tinnitus, or ringing in the ears, is a warning signal. If you notice this symptom after taking aspirin, beware. Consult an otologist if you must continue to take aspirin for chronic pain, and have your hearing checked regularly. There are other nonprescription pills that can be taken for pain and do not contain aspirin. Seek and *follow* your physician's advice in this important matter!

Quinine is also known to produce toxic effects on hearing, and the sulfa drugs and antihistamines have this consequence too for some people.

Are antibiotics dangerous to hearing? Besides causing the middle-ear problem of "glue ear" discussed in Chapter 3, certain antibiotics have been indicted as producers of sensori-neural hearing loss in susceptible individuals. These include dihydrostreptomycin, kanamycin, streptomycin, neomycin, vancomycin. You should never take these drugs unless they are necessary to save your life. A big problem now is that new antibiotics are being developed so rapidly that they may be used before doctors become aware of their possible bad effects on hearing. If your doctor prescribes an antibiotic for you, be sure to ask him whether or not it has been thoroughly tested for toxic effects on the hearing mechanism. You have a right to ask that question, and most doctors won't resent your concern. After all, it's *your* hearing that may hang in the balance.

Can smoking cause sensori-neural hearing loss? We have seen in Chapter 3 that smoking can cause middle-ear problems resulting in conductive impairment. Now there is evidence that heavy smoking can also damage blood vessels and cells in the cochlea of the inner ear. Andrews University audiologist Stephen Prescod, reporting on clinical research, says there is a definite link between heavy smoking and loss of hearing. "Smoking can affect one's hearing in much the same way that aging does," says Prescod. "Those smoking twenty or more cigarettes a day can expect enough loss in sensitivity to both high and low frequencies to impair understanding of normal speech." He goes on to report that "though smokers may not be aware of hearing problems for years, the damage is nonetheless taking place."[8] Lung cancer, heart disease, hearing loss—how much of ourselves are we willing to risk playing cigarette roulette?

What about sensori-neural hearing loss caused by the process of aging? Newby names the aging process as the most common cause of sensori-neural hearing impairment. "The study of large samples of the population demonstrates that the process starts at about the age of twenty and becomes increasingly noticeable with each succeeding decade."[9] So if your otologist or audiologist tells you that your hearing loss is caused by aging and you're only fifty years old, don't be insulted. Remember that this deterioration begins at age twenty. A study by John F. Corso indicates that hearing loss due to aging usually affects the higher frequencies first and that women tend to have better hearing than men at all ages.[10] Of course, not all old people are hard of hearing. Though the problem used to be termed *senile deafness,* this is not an appropriate name for it. Many people who find their hearing ability slipping with age are very alert mentally, while some oldsters who are regrettably senile have excellent hearing. The technical term for loss of hearing caused by aging is *presbycusis.*

What causes this loss of hearing that comes with aging? It's usually due to a deterioration of the auditory nerve fibers in the cochlea. Sometimes it's associated with high blood pressure and hardening of the arteries, but this is not always the case. People who are exposed to an excessive amount of noise during their working years are likely to develop presbycusis at an earlier age than most. In addition to these physical factors, Canfield reports that "a progressive hearing loss often occurs in people whose lives are devoid of a feeling of security and faith for some reason."[11] Some people hate to admit that their hearing is failing, because they associate hearing loss with old age, so they put off seeking help. This is about as sensible as refusing to go on a diet because you hate to admit that you're gaining weight. But, just as it's a lot easier to do something about ten extra pounds than thirty, it's much easier to help a person whose hearing loss is just beginning than one who has waited until he can no longer understand what people are saying.

The term sensori-neural hearing loss refers to problems occurring in the inner ear and the auditory nerve. There is another kind of auditory disorder that results from interference in the nerve pathways of the brain *beyond* the auditory nerve. This is termed *central deafness.*

What are the causes of central deafness? Causes include brain tumor, vascular disturbances in the brain, cerebral hemorrhage, and brain damage from such traumas as birth injuries, gunshot wounds, and skull fractures. The person with this kind of hearing problem has trouble understanding the meaning of words even though he actually *hears* sounds normally.

Brian, the young man I told you about at the beginning of the chapter who fractured his skull in an automobile accident, suffered from central deafness. He had had hearing tests in school, so verbal explanation wasn't essential to his ability to respond to pure-tone hearing testing, and he did respond normally. Even though the tests showed that his hearing was good, he still couldn't understand speech because of the brain damage caused by his skull fracture.

Central deafness is a neurological disorder rather than a true hearing defect and therefore should be treated by a neurologist or neuropsychiatrist. It is usually accompanied by problems in understanding and using language, and this requires help from a speech pathologist.

Is it possible for a person to really believe that he is deaf, even though his hearing is actually normal? Surprisingly, yes. This belongs in the category of *functional hearing loss.* In such cases, there is no organic (physical) abnormality that would cause loss of hearing. Functional hearing disorders fall into two groups: (1) hysterical, or psychogenic, deafness, in which the patient really believes he has a genuine hearing loss; and (2) malingering, in which the individual is trying to fake a hearing loss.

Persons who suffer from psychogenic hearing loss often have an unconscious desire to escape from some situation in their lives that has become intolerable for them. They are not faking. They are truly convinced that they cannot hear. Remember Susan, the girl who cried "I can't hear anything" after she was hit on the ear by a volleyball? I think you'd be interested in her case. She was brought to me for testing when I was a public school speech and hearing therapist. The first thing I noticed was that, although she "couldn't hear" what I said to her, she spoke in a perfectly normal voice. There was no increase in volume, as there would have been in a person who had suddenly become truly deaf. Then, too, there was no expression of straining to hear or searching for visual cues as I spoke to her. Instead, her eyes wandered *away* from my face as I spoke, giving the distinct impression that she was *not* trying to hear. In fact, she was unconsciously trying not to hear. Still, she answered some of my questions and followed my directions in preparing for the audiometric test. But she showed no response whatever to any of the tones, even at the highest level of loudness. I suggested psychiatric counseling. During the course of therapy, Susan gradually opened up and finally revealed the following incident.

One afternoon, while her mother was away from home, an insurance man had come to the door asking for a policy her father had told him to pick up. Susan found it for him in the family safe. After the man left, Susan went back to close up the safe and began looking through some of the family papers stored there. What she found was shattering. Buried under a pile of papers was her parents' marriage certificate, dated in January of the year Susan was born. Susan's birthday was in May. To add to the shock, she then discovered her mother's passport, which showed she had been in Europe at the time Susan was conceived. The girl had often heard her mother speak of that trip to Europe, and she knew that her father had never been out of the United States. The truth suddenly caved in on her—not only had she been conceived out of wedlock, but the man she'd been calling Dad wasn't even her natural father! Of course, she couldn't bear to say anything about her crushing discovery to anyone, least of all to her parents. So she bound the wound up inside of her, where it festered for several days until she was offered an escape. When the volleyball hit her on the ear and her phys. ed. teacher asked if she could still hear, Susan's unconscious mind grabbed at this excuse to partially shut out a world that had grown painfully hostile. I'm glad to tell you that, through continued counseling, Susan was able to face and finally accept her life situation, and her hearing returned to normal.

But what about people who intentionally fake a hearing loss? Those who do this are called *malingerers,* and they know perfectly well that their hearing is normal. Or, in some cases, they may have a slight hearing loss that they decide to capitalize on by faking a more severe loss.

Why? Usually, they are out after disability payments for injury on the job, or a medical discharge from the service, or some other mercenary advantage. They may try feigning hearing loss to avoid the draft or to get out of some other unpleasant task. It is not difficult for the experienced audiologist to detect malingering. Special testing techniques have been devised just for this purpose, and these tests are good detectives. Of course, I know that you aren't included in this group, or you wouldn't be reading a book on how to cope with hearing loss. Still, a description of the causes of hearing impairment wouldn't be complete without some reference to functional hearing loss.

In Chapters 3 and 4, I have discussed conductive, sensori-neural, central, and functional hearing impairment. In order to make the distinctions clear, I have considered only "pure" conductive and "pure" sensori-neural losses. It is not unusual, though, for patients to have a combination of conductive and sensori-neural impairment. For instance, a person with otosclerosis may have, in addition to his middle-ear problem, some inner-ear or nerve deterioration. An elderly person with sensori-neural loss may also develop a wax plug in the ear canal. In Chapter 6, I'll give you some sample audiograms that will help to further clarify the differences among the various types of hearing loss.

Again I need to remind you that these descriptions of the symptoms and causes of hearing loss are not intended as diagnostic tools. Only your physician or otologist can diagnose your hearing problem. Consult him at the first sign of hearing loss, and then reread these chapters. They may help to clarify for you, at your leisure, some of the things your medical specialist has told you about your hearing problem.

Is it true that nothing can be done to help the person with a sensori-neural hearing loss? Emphatically not! Sure, people with conductive losses stand a much better chance of being helped by medical and surgical treatment, though *some* types of sensori-neural loss do also respond to treatment. But even if your loss is permanent, you, too, can break through that sound barrier, through help in auditory training, speech retraining, lipreading, and/or manual communication. (See Chapters 9, 10, and 11.) You *can* learn to use a hearing aid (Chapters 7 and 8) and you *can* adjust to the social, psychological, and family problems you face. (Chapters 12 and 15) Your hearing loss can shut you away from the world only if you refuse to open the door.

5

Will medical or surgical treatment help me?

Have you ever made any of the following statements, to yourself or to others?

"I don't have *time* to see a doctor about my hearing difficulties."

"I get by. I've learned to live with my hearing loss. Why should I rock the boat?"

"I can't afford an expensive operation or involved treatment."

"My loss isn't all that bad. Now *Mrs. Smith* across the street, *she* should have something done, but I can hear a lot better than she can."

"I've got the kind of hearing loss that can't be helped. I'll just have to put up with it."

"Maybe the doctor will suggest an operation. Frankly, the thought scares me."

"If my hearing gets *really* bad, I'll see if something can be done, but not now."

"I'm probably too old to be helped, anyway."

"So I've got a hearing loss. Big deal. At least I'm not blind or crippled."

"Hearing loss means old age. I'm only forty. Can I help it if people don't speak clearly these days?"

Do you recognize yourself in any of these statements? If so, you may be cheating yourself out of the chance for better hearing. If you lost $500, would you refuse to look for it because you're getting by all right without it, or because you didn't have time to look, or because there's a chance you might not find it even if you did search? Good hearing is worth immeasurably more than $500. Think about it.

True, some people *do* have hearing impairments that can't be

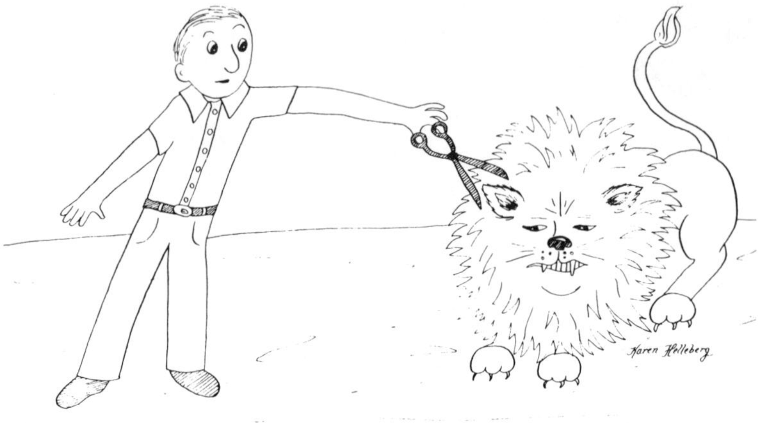

Figure 5.1. In medieval times, a lion's right ear was said to cure deafness. All you had to do was cut if off, hold it over the afflicted person's ear, and say the magic words.

helped by medicine or surgery. If you're one of these, your doctor will tell you so, and he'll refer you to someone who can help you through nonmedical methods of aural rehabilitation. But many people with hearing losses *can* be helped to regain all or part of their hearing. Maybe you're one of them.

If you had been living in the twelfth or thirteenth century, you might have listened to Saint Albertus Magnus, who wrote, "Lion's brain, if eaten, causes madness, but remedies deafness if inserted in the ear with some strong oil." Or you might have followed the treatment recommended by Saint Hildegard of Bingen, who said that "deafness may be remedied by cutting off a lion's right ear and holding it over the patient's ear just long enough to say, 'Hear, *Adimacus,* by the living god of the keen virtue of a lion's hearing,' and that 'the heart of a weasel, dried and placed with wax in the ear, benefits headache or deafness.'"[1] I'm sure you're not going to go on a lion hunt or rush out and kill a weasel. In case you're not in the mood for lion's ears or brains or weasels' hearts, medical science has developed techniques that are much less repulsive and certainly more effective.

In this chapter, we'll talk about some of the treatments available for various ear conditions. Bear in mind, though, that this section of the book is definitely *not* a self-help manual. Not one of the treatments discussed here can be safely self-administered. Not even wax removal.

How does the doctor remove ear wax? He may do it by irrigating the canal with water injected from a syringe.

Why can't I do this myself? By examining your ears with an instrument called a speculum, the doctor can make sure *all* of the excess wax is removed. If you tried to do the job yourself, some of the wax plug might remain in your ear, and the injected water would cause that residue to swell, creating further problems. Also, there may be other ear-canal problems in addition to the wax plug that need treatment.

What if irrigating doesn't get rid of the plug? Then the doctor will have to use instruments to remove it. Occasionally, wax that has become impacted with a mass of skin has to be removed under local anesthetic, but this doesn't happen very often.

How are skin irritations of the ear canal treated? Your doctor may apply medication to the swollen or sensitive area. He may ask you to refrain from swimming until the condition heals. In some chronic cases in which the canal has become narrowed, he may gradually enlarge the opening by inserting polythene or rubber tubes in successively larger sizes.[2]

So far, we've been talking about treatments for outer-ear problems. Now let's turn our attention to middle-ear conditions that may cause hearing loss.

As I explained in Chapter 2, the eustachian tube, leading from the middle ear into the throat area behind the nose, helps to equalize the air pressure in the middle ear. Sometimes, though, this tube becomes blocked.

What can be done for a blocked eustachian tube? The doctor will probably first direct his attention to clearing up any swelling of the nose-throat area that may be causing the blockage. After the swelling subsides, it will take about a week to ten days for the eustachian tube to return to normal. The physician may decide to help it along by inserting a tube through the nostril and forcing a small amount of air into the middle ear. Sometimes tonsils and/or adenoids interfere with the action of the eustachian tube and have to be removed to relieve the pressure. This usually clears up middle-ear problems related to such blockage.

In what ways are middle ear infections (otitis media) treated? Antibiotics are often prescribed. Also, as I explained in Chapter 3, these infections often cause fluid to accumulate in the middle ear. If there's danger of the eardrum breaking from the pressure of this fluid, the physician will probably make a small incision in the drum so the fluid can drain out. When recurring ear infections are caused by enlarged tonsils and adenoids, removal may be recommended.

Why not just wait to see if the eardrum breaks by itself? The small, clean slit the doctor makes is much less likely to result in permanent damage to the eardrum. A drum that ruptures by itself may heal improperly and leave scar tissue or a permanent perforation, or hole, in this important membrane. Besides causing hearing loss, a perforated drum is a threat to the middle ear.

Is there anything that can be done about a scarred or perforated drum, once the damage is done? Sometimes healing is induced by applying an irritating solution to the edges of the perforation, or by skin grafting. An "artificial eardrum" (prosthesis) may be placed over the opening. When the perforation is sealed by one of the above methods, hearing usually improves or returns to normal, and the constant danger of middle-ear infection is reduced.

How is "glue ear" treated? In cases of chronic middle-ear infection in which the fluid has become thickened and "gluey," it may be necessary for the otologist to insert a small tube into the middle ear through a small incision in the eardrum. After removing the fluid by suction, he leaves the tube in place for a time. This lets air into the middle ear so that healing can occur.

What about surgery for otosclerosis? As you may remember from our discussion in Chapter 3, the stirrup bone of the middle ear sometimes becomes fixed at the point where it touches the membrane leading into the inner ear. The condition that causes this is called otosclerosis. This impairment usually appears in the late teens or early twenties and seems to run in families. Not every patient who has otosclerosis can benefit from surgery. If the disease has spread into the cochlea of the inner ear, then surgery may not help much. Before the otologist decides to operate, he performs a series of careful diagnostic tests to determine whether or not surgery is advisable.

If surgery is advised, what does this involve? Several different techniques have been devised for correcting or improving this condition. The three that are best known are stapes mobilization, fenestration, and stapedectomy.

"*Stapes mobilization* consists of laying back the eardrum and manipulating the bones of the middle ear with an instrument . . . until the stapes (stirrup bone) is broken free from the otosclerotic growth that surrounds it."[3] If this procedure is successful, patients may experience a dramatic return of hearing, which sometimes occurs right on the operating table.

In the *fenestration* operation, the surgeon removes the head of the hammer and anvil bones and makes a new window to the inner ear. This causes the sound vibrations to bypass the oval window, which isn't working anyway because of the fixation of the stirrup bone. The fenestration operation cannot restore a patient's hearing to normal because it makes the middle-ear bone chain nonfunctional. This operation is not used very often anvmore

The *stapedectomy* technique was developed in 1956 by J. J. Shea, Jr., and has virtually replaced the fenestration and stapes mobilization procedures. In this operation, the fixated bone (stapes) is completely removed and an artificial "bone" is inserted in its place. The new "bone" connects the anvil (middle bone of the chain) with the oval window, which has been repaired. Most surgeons use only a local anesthetic for this surgery, and most patients are ready to leave the hospital the next day. If you have a stapedectomy operation, you may actually notice a sudden recovery of hearing, even during surgery. Don't be upset, though, if this improvement seems to dwindle during the recovery period. It usually takes one to two weeks for healing, and there is normally a decline in hearing acuity during this period. About a month after you've had the operation, your hearing should be at its maximum, though it may continue to improve slightly during the next six months. According to Harold Schuknecht, excellent results are obtained in ninety percent of carefully done stapedectomy operations.[4] The rate of failure for the operation is low, side effects are very rare, and "95% of the patients who have been periodically checked have maintained their improved hearing."[5]

David S. Akens, whose hearing was restored by this operation, told of his experience in an article for *Mature Years* magazine, which was later reprinted in his book, *Loss of Hearing and You.* Like many people, he was at first reluctant to seek help. His wife had to use some of her cleverest feminine wiles to get him to the otologist. Then, when the doctor recommended surgery, Akens groped about for an excuse to escape it but finally agreed to the operation. The result?

> Exactly seven days after the operation, I heard our air conditioner for the first time.

> "Helen!" I exclaimed, "the air conditioner's broken! It sounds like a freight train!" And never had I heard such a great sound![6]

If your otologist recommends a stapedectomy operation for you, by all means, *have* it!

Reconstructive surgery is also performed when the other two bones of the middle ear have been damaged by injury or growths. Surgery to eliminate infection in the mastoid bone and preserve hearing is now possible. In some cases in which previous surgery for mastoid infection had created a hearing loss, it is possible to improve hearing by reconstructive surgery.

What can be done, medically, for other causes of conductive impairment? Often, treatment of the contributing causes will improve or restore hearing. For instance, if the otologist feels that your hearing loss is caused by sinus trouble or allergy, he'll no doubt refer you to a specialist in the appropriate area. If your jaws don't fit together properly because of crooked or missing teeth, this may cause a hearing problem. An orthodontist should be consulted. The solution to hearing problems caused by smoking should be obvious, though not necessarily easy to accomplish. If you can't seem to stop smoking, ask your doctor for suggestions to help you break the habit.

Is sensori-neural hearing loss hopeless? No. It's true that *most* cases of sensori-neural impairment are not, at the present time, responsive to medical treatment, and the "miracle" operations that restore hearing to people with middle-ear problems won't do you any good if yours is an inner-ear or nerve problem. But, as Herman Wallenfels points out, "Nerve deafness should never be called 'hopeless' in an out-of-hand manner. After all, we can lose quite a few of those one hundred thousand nerve endings and still have a workable number left over."[7] In this residual hearing—the hearing you still have left—lies your hope and your chance for breaking through that "sound barrier" to more effective communication. If you spend your energies concentrating on your *loss,* rather than on making the most effective use of what hearing you *have,* you're like the person who sees the glass as half empty instead of half full. If your otologist tells you that you have a permanent sensori-neural hearing loss, your number one priority should be to do everything in your power to conserve the hearing you still have. I'll make some specific suggestions for this in Chapter 11. Your second priority will be to learn to *use* your hearing and your other senses to your own best advantage, through auditory training and lipreading.

What types of sensori-neural impairments do respond to treatment? If you suffer from Meniere's disease, various treatments are available, ranging from treatment for allergy to use of ultrasonic vibrations. This disease is also subject to natural remissions, or improvements, and new treatments are being developed for alleviation of its symptoms. Have confidence in your otologist. He knows what treatments are most likely to help you.

In cases of sudden, severe hearing loss due to interruption of the blood supply to the cochlea, "the prompt administration of a vasodilator (blood-vessel relaxer), perhaps in combination with an anticoagulant (a drug that reduces blood clotting), will sometimes result in a dramatic restoration of hearing."[8]

Roeser, Campbell, and Daly cite evidence from two case histories of deafness from meningitis to support their contention that "although it occurs rarely, some patients recover auditory function following meningitic deafness."[9] Since these researchers also note that "typically, the hearing loss [from meningitis] is permanent, severe to profound, bilateral, and sensori-neural," I see their findings as evidence that there is sometimes a crack in the slammed door of sensori-neural hearing impairment.

Is surgery ever performed in cases of sensori-neural hearing loss? If the loss is caused by a tumor pressing on the nerve fibers, it may be possible to remove the tumor or to reduce it by radiation therapy to prevent further loss.

What about prevention of sensori-neural loss? Of course, preventive measures won't restore the hearing you've already lost, but they may prevent *further* loss, and they may save your *children* from having hearing impairments. Genetic counseling prior to pregnancy, immunization of the potential mother against rubella and other infectious diseases, abstinence from drugs during pregnancy, careful control of the Rh blood factor, and the best possible obstetrical care can prevent many cases of congenital hearing impairment.

If you already have a hearing loss, you'll want to see your doctor at the first sign of any infectious disease, protect your ears from noise, avoid taking any drugs that are suspected of causing hearing loss, and, if you are a heavy smoker or a "coffee addict," cut down on your intake or stop altogether for a while. Your hearing loss *may* have nothing to do with your coffee habit, but we do know that, in some cases, there is a correlation, possibly due to allergy. I have an aunt in Kansas who has a hearing loss that was becoming rapidly and progressively more severe. She was a heavy coffee drinker. Two years ago, her otologist advised her to stop drinking coffee. Although her hearing has not improved, her loss has *not increased at all* in the two years since she stopped drinking coffee.

Can central deafness be treated? Remedial measures may be taken, depending on the *cause* of the central impairment. Since this is a neurological problem, details about treatment are outside the scope of this book.

What about functional hearing loss? In cases where emotional problems are the cause of the hearing loss, normal hearing may be restored through counseling and/or psychotherapy.

In this chapter, I have touched on some of the more common medical and surgical treatments available to the hard of hearing. Obviously, a book of this nature demands some oversimplification because most of us lack the medical background necessary to understand the technical details of these procedures. If you want to do further reading in this area, I recommend the references that follow.

An article in the August, 1975, issue of *Changing Times* magazine asserts that, while hearing loss is this country's most prevalent physical disorder, "yet by a conservative estimate, no more than 25% of the Americans who need help for hearing problems have received it."[10] Please. Don't be one of the seventy-five percent who suffer in silence! Seek help *now*.

6

What do I need to know about hearing testing, audiograms, and the degree of handicap caused by my loss?

What kinds of hearing tests are most accurate? Am I deaf or just hard of hearing? What is my percentage of hearing loss? Is my loss conductive or sensori-neural? Will a hearing aid help me? How severe is my hearing handicap? What can I learn about my loss by studying my audiogram? How does my age affect my ability to adjust to my hearing handicap? What if I have impaired hearing in only one ear?

People with defective hearing want and have a *right* to know the answers to questions such as these. Yet they often hesitate to ask because they feel it's an imposition on the time of the busy professional people who examine them. But you and I, as reader and writer, have as much time to spend together as you want to take. In this chapter, I'll try to answer some of your questions about such things as: what distinguishes the "deaf" from the "hard of hearing;" what to expect when you go for a hearing test; how to interpret your own audiogram; how your loss affects your understanding of speech; the degree of handicap caused by a monaural (one ear) hearing loss; how the *pattern* of your loss affects the usability of your hearing; and other questions about *hearing evaluation* that may have been churning around in your mind.

Where do we draw the line between the terms "deaf" and "hard of hearing"? Actually, there are *very few* people who have no hearing at all. Even those who are considered profoundly deaf generally have some residual hearing. So the distinction between one person who is classified as deaf and another who is hard of hearing is based on the *usefulness* of the hearing that remains. A person whose loss is severe enough that his hearing is not usable for the ordinary purposes of life is considered deaf. On the other hand, an individual whose hearing is defective but still usable is considered hard of hearing. This latter group includes those whose hearing is functional only with the help of a hearing aid as well as those who have some usable hearing without amplification. There are a number of factors that help determine how useful a person's hearing is, including *amount* of loss, *pattern* of loss, and *age* of the patient at the time the loss occurred. We'll discuss these elements later in the chapter. First, let's talk about hearing tests.

Can hearing be tested accurately without electrical machines? Several tests performed without an audiometer can spot *gross* abnormalities in hearing. Your family physician may, for instance, hold his watch up to your ear and gradually move it away, asking you to let him know when you can no longer hear it ticking. Or he may drop a large coin on his desk and ask if you hear a ringing sound or just a thud. He may have you stand across the room from him, with first one ear plugged and then the other, and ask you to repeat what he says. These tests are better than nothing, and they *can* be helpful in determining whether or not you need further testing. They can't, though, reveal anything about the *type* or *pattern* of loss, and they can yield only a rough estimate of the degree of loss. Then, too, because the testing conditions are difficult to control, you may be able to "pass" such a test even though you have a moderate loss.

What about tuning-fork tests? Tuning forks are Y-shaped metal instruments that emit tones of specific frequencies, or pitches, when set in vibration. For testing hearing, a vibrating fork may be held close to the external ear or placed on the mastoid bone behind the ear. Tuning-fork tests can be useful in differentiating between conductive and sensori-neural hearing loss, and they can give some estimate of the *amount* of sensori-neural loss. They are more useful for determining the *type* of loss than the *degree* of loss.

What is a pure-tone audiometer? It's an instrument that produces, electrically, tones similar to those made by the tuning fork. Each tone generated consists of a single frequency, so that's why it's called a *pure-tone* audiometer. Modern audiometers usually produce the following frequencies, from lowest to highest: 125, 250, 500, 750, 1,000, 1,500, 2,000, 3,000, 4,000, 6,000, and 8,000 Hz. (Hz, or hertz, as you may remember, means the same as cycles per second and refers to the number of complete sound wave cycles that occur in a second of time. The higher the number of cycles per second, or hertz, the higher pitched the tone is.)

Besides being capable of producing tones of different *frequen-*

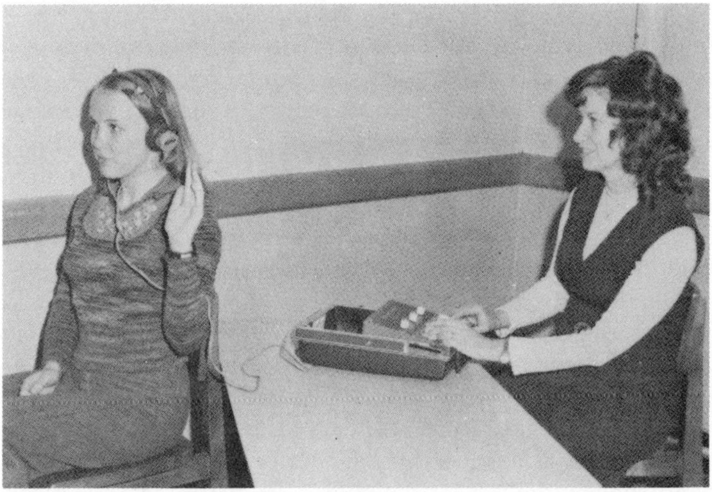

Figure 6.1. A portable audiometer offers a convenient way to test hearing.

cies, the audiometer can also present each of these tones at various degrees of loudness, or decibels. Zero decibels of loudness on the audiometer represents the level at which the average normal ear can just barely hear a particular tone. So if the examiner has to turn the loudness up to fifty decibels before you can hear a certain tone, he would say that you have a fifty-decibel loss for that frequency.

When you have your hearing tested audiometrically, the tones are delivered to one ear and then the other, first through headphones and then through a bone-conduction vibrator that is placed on the bone behind your ear. If facilities are available, the tester may also have you listen for tones coming into the sound booth over a loudspeaker, without using headphones or a bone-conduction vibrator. This is called *free-field* testing, and it allows him to determine your hearing level when you are using both ears at once.

Is it really necessary to test with the bone-conduction vibrator as well as the headphones? Yes! Unless the test with the headphones has shown your hearing to be normal, it is very important that you also have a test by bone conduction.

Why? In air-conduction testing, the sound passes from the earphones through the outer, middle, and inner ear to the auditory nerve. Obviously, if you hear the test sound normally this way, all the parts of the hearing mechanism must be working properly. *But,* if this air conduction test (with earphones) shows that you have a hearing loss, the trouble *may* be only in the outer or middle ear. The bone conduction test, with the vibrator placed on the bone behind your ear, *sends the tones directly into your inner ear.* It's entirely possible that your hearing by bone conduction may be normal, indicating that the inner ear and nerve are undamaged. If so, it's obvious that your problem lies in the outer or middle ear. It is not uncommon for people to purchase expensive hearing aids only to find out later that their hearing losses were caused by something as simple as a wax plug! That's why most reputable hearing aid dealers prefer to have you see your physician or otologist before you buy a hearing aid.

Remember: Unless your hearing is *normal,* your hearing examination is *not complete* without a bone conduction test.

What is masking? Many people who are hard of hearing have a greater degree of loss in one ear than in the other. Sometimes, when the poorer ear is being tested, the better ear picks up some of the sound, making the test for the poorer ear invalid. This is especially likely to happen in bone-conduction testing, though if the difference between the ears is great enough, such crossover may also occur in air-conduction testing. To prevent crossover, the examiner introduces a *masking noise* into the better ear while testing the poorer one. Several types of masking noise are available, but the one most commonly used is "white noise," which sounds kind of like the audio on a TV set before the station comes on the air.

What is a speech audiometer? While a pure-tone audiometer transmits single-frequency sounds to the ear, a speech audiometer transmits words or sentences to the listener. The test is used to determine how well you are able to discriminate among the different sounds of speech. If you have a speech discrimination test, you will probably be seated in a sound booth, and the examiner will be in a separate room. He either will speak the test words or sentences directly into a microphone or will send *taped* speech sounds through the audiometer to you. In either case, the examiner will be able to accurately control the loudness of the speech sounds that he directs to one ear at a time, or to both ears, through earphones or by loudspeaker. He'll ask you to *identify* the words you hear, by repeating them back to him, by checking them off on a multiple-choice list, by writing them down, or by answering questions.

What's the purpose of a speech discrimination test? *Hearing* really has two meanings. One refers to the ability to be *aware of the presence of sound,* and the pure-tone audiometer checks this. It isn't enough, though, to be able to barely hear pure tones. If your hearing is to be usable for communication, you also need to be able to hear well enough to *attach meaning to speech sounds.* The speech audiometric test can reveal some very important information about your hearing, including:

1. *Speech reception threshold.* This is the level of loudness at which you can just barely understand speech. It is established by determining the amount of amplification necessary for you to correctly identify fifty percent of the test words. This measurement helps to determine how usable your residual hearing is for communication purposes. The score, when compared with your pure-tone test results, may help with diagnosis of your hearing problem. If the results of the two tests are inconsistent, this fact may help the otologist in diagnosing certain types of sensori-neural loss, or it may suggest that psychological factors are involved in the hearing problem.

2. *Most comfortable level of loudness.* This measurement is especially valuable for determining the amount of amplification a hearing-aid candidate should have. If you have a hearing aid stashed away in the dresser drawer because you "couldn't stand the noise," this measurement and the next one might help with your adjustment problem. See if there is someone in your area who has the equipment for testing your hearing by speech audiometry.

3. *Tolerance level.* This is the level at which speech becomes *uncomfortably loud* for you. The normal ear should be able to tolerate speech at hearing levels of 90 to 100 decibels without discomfort. But remember the *recruitment* factor we talked about in Chapter 4? It's that rapid increase in the sensation of loudness that occurs in many people who have sensori-neural losses. Through speech audiometry, the examiner can determine, first of all, how loud speech needs to be for you to understand it, and second, how much *more* loudness you can take without becoming uncomfortable. Then he can arrange for your hearing aid to be set somewhere in between these two measurements. As I mentioned earlier, your tolerance level can probably be increased through auditory training, but it is necessary to know what

that level is to begin with, so that the increase can be made gradually. (See Chapter 10.)

4. *Speech discrimination ability.* This is a gauge of your ability to distinguish among the various vowel and consonant sounds that make up the language. It's designed for the "I-hear-you-but-I-don't-understand-you" people. If you often misunderstand because you've mistaken a word for one that rhymes with it, this test will help to pinpoint your problem sounds.

Incidentally, if you have difficulty this way, you're in good company. Most people with sensori-neural losses belong to the "club"! Let me tell you about the case of the too-obedient son. The mother of a young client of mine told me about the time she invited the family next door over for a backyard picnic. Before the guests arrived, she warned her hard-of-hearing son to try to *please* Sally—the neighbors' young, good-looking daughter. A few minutes after the visitors got there, he started putting ice cubes down Sally's back, tickling her, untying her shoes, etc. His embarrassed mother couldn't understand what had happened to her usually polite son—until she realized that he thought she'd said to try to *tease* Sally! If you misunderstand similar-sounding words, I'll bet you could tell some equally embarrassing tales.

Is it really necessary to have your hearing tested by speech audiometry as well as by pure tone? Let's say this: Speech audiometry is an extremely useful tool in planning for your aural rehabilitation. I'd advise anyone who considers purchasing a hearing aid to insist on having a speech discrimination test if at all possible. If your hearing aid dealer doesn't have facilities for this, try to locate an audiologist or speech and hearing clinic that does. The tests will improve your chances of getting an aid that suits you well, and having the scores available will help the therapist who works with you on auditory training. If speech audiometric equipment is simply not available in your area, there are certain practical tests of hearing aid performance that can be used (as a second choice) in place of it. We'll go into these in detail in Chapter 7.

Is it necessary to have a sound-treated room or sound booth for testing hearing? Some people have argued that, since we live in a world of sound, testing for hearing aids should be done in a "normal" environment instead of in a sound booth. This argument ignores the *purpose* of testing. The otologist, *who is the only person capable of*

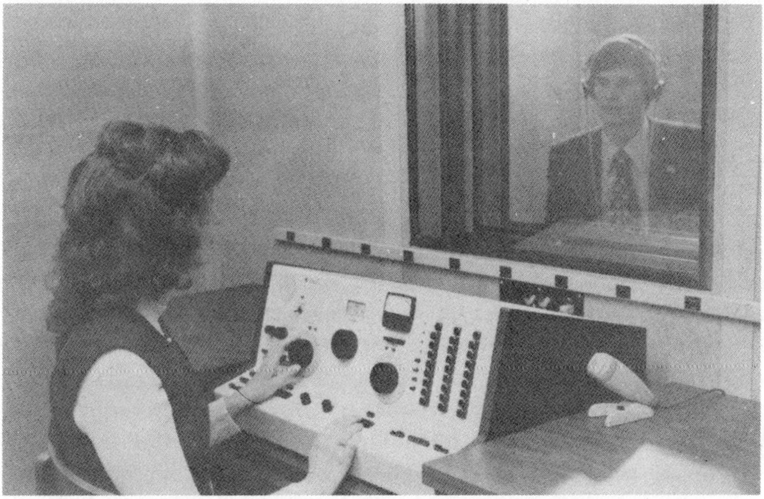

Figure 6.2. This two-room sound suite and console audiometer at Kearney State College provides the most accurate type of testing situation.

making a medical diagnosis of your hearing problem, needs some specific information about your ability to respond to various sounds. He may do his own testing, or he may rely on test results provided him by an audiologist. Background noise of any kind can distort the results of your hearing test, and misleading information may therefore result. The audiologist or speech and hearing clinician who will help with your aural rehabilitation also needs accurate information that can only be provided by tests conducted under optimum conditions. Having your hearing tested in a special sound-treated room is the best way to ensure accuracy at this crucial stage in the evaluation process. Later, when it's time to make a decision about a particular hearing aid, you'll want to make additional tests under various conditions of noise outside a sound booth. (More about that in Chapter 7.)

What is an audiogram? It's a type of graph on which the examiner records the results of your hearing test. Most audiograms have the numbers that represent frequencies (from 125 Hz to 8,000 Hz) marked along the horizontal plane—going across the page—and the hearing level in decibels (loudness) listed vertically—up and down the page. (See Figure 6.3) The level of loudness at which you can *just* *barely hear* a tone is called your *threshold.* As the examiner determines your threshold for each tone, he places a mark on the audiogram at the point where the line for that level of loudness intersects the line for the frequency being tested. Red markings are used for the right ear and black or blue for the left. The symbols for air-conduction testing (that is, tests performed with earphones) are: *O* for the right ear and *X* for the left. An arrow pointing to the left represents the bone-conduction threshold for the left ear, while the right-ear bone-conduction score is shown by an arrow pointing to the right. This may sound confusing as you read it, but if you'll study the form and key in Figure 6.3, I'm sure you'll be able to understand the audiograms and explanations that follow. The symbols for each ear are usually connected by a line of the appropriate color, so that the pattern of the loss becomes obvious at a glance. To avoid confusion, bone-conduction markings are either connected by a broken line or not connected at all.

The audiogram shown in Figure 6.4 represents normal hearing. As you can see, the symbols are all on the zero-decibel line. Actually, most people with normal hearing have some variation in their ability to hear different frequencies, so a "normal" audiogram might have some markings above the zero line and some a bit below but still fall within normal limits.

Figure 6.5 shows the audiogram of a person with a conductive hearing loss. Notice that the *X* and *O* symbols, which represent air-conduction results, show about a fifty-decibel loss in both ears. *But,* the symbols < >, representing bone-conduction testing (vibrator on mastoid bone), are in the normal range. Since these tones are transmitted directly to the inner ear without having to go through the outer or middle ear, we can see that this person's inner ear and nerve are normal. Obviously, the problem must be somewhere in the outer or middle ear. Only the frequencies from 500 Hz to 4,000 Hz are generally tested by bone conduction because most audiometers are not capable of producing enough intensity at the very high and very low frequencies through the vibrator to allow for accurate testing. The pattern of the loss shown in Figure 6.5 is relatively *flat.* The individual's threshold for all frequencies is about the same. This is typical of most conductive impairments. If your audiogram is similar to this one, your otologist may be able to correct, or at least greatly improve, your hearing, medically or surgically. If not, a hearing aid will help you immeasurably.

Figure 6.6 depicts a typical sensori-neural impairment. The

Figure 6.3. AUDIOGRAM

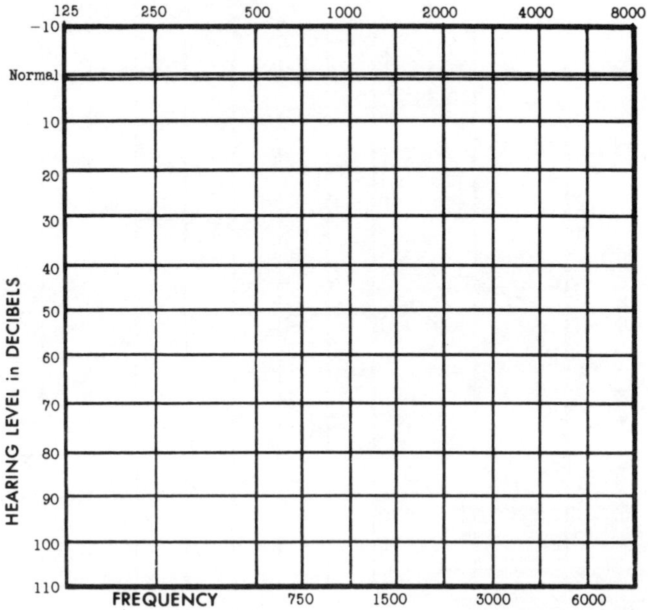

Figure 6.4. AUDIOGRAM

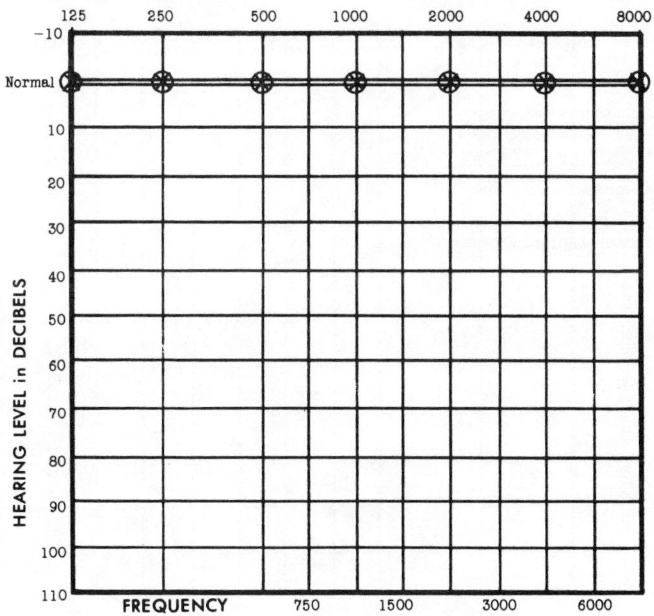

AC = testing by air conduction
BC = testing by bone conduction vibrator

		AC	AC (masked)	BC	BC (masked)
Right	Red*	○	△	>	▷
Left	Blue*	×	□	<	◁

*Color not shown in these audiograms.

Figure 6.5. AUDIOGRAM

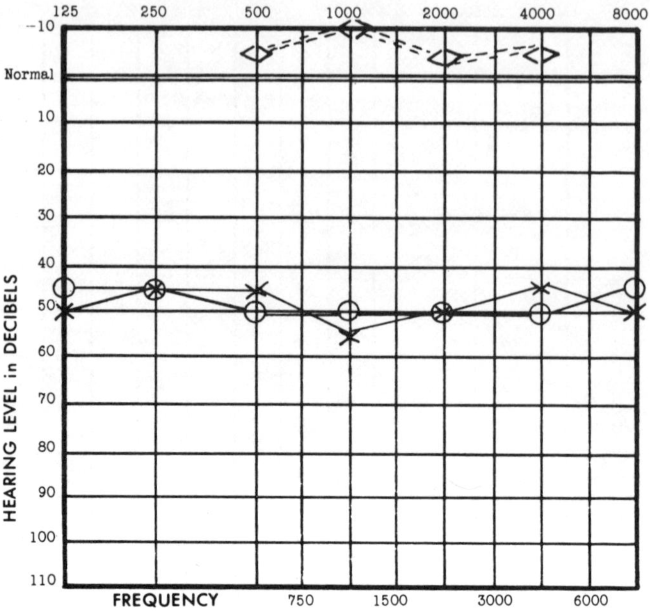

Figure 6.6. AUDIOGRAM

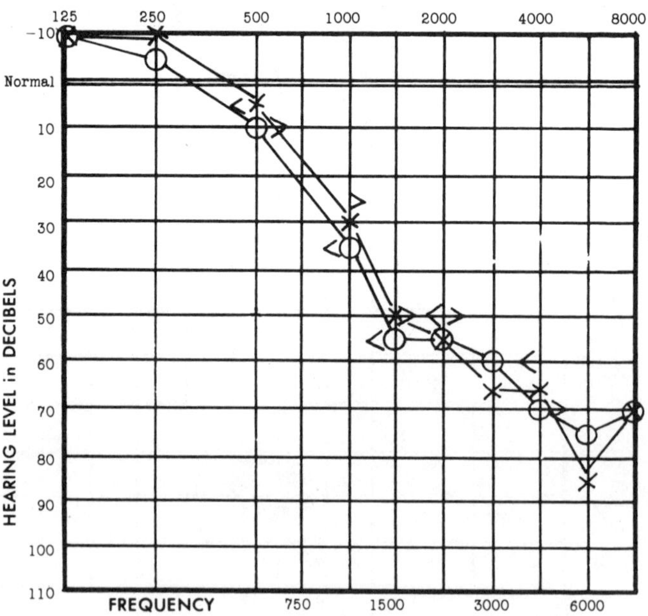

AC = testing by air conduction
BC = testing by bone conduction vibrator

		AC	AC (masked)	BC	BC (masked)
Right	Red*	○	△	>	▷
Left	Blue*	×	□	<	◁

*Color not shown in these audiograms.

Figure 6.7. AUDIOGRAM

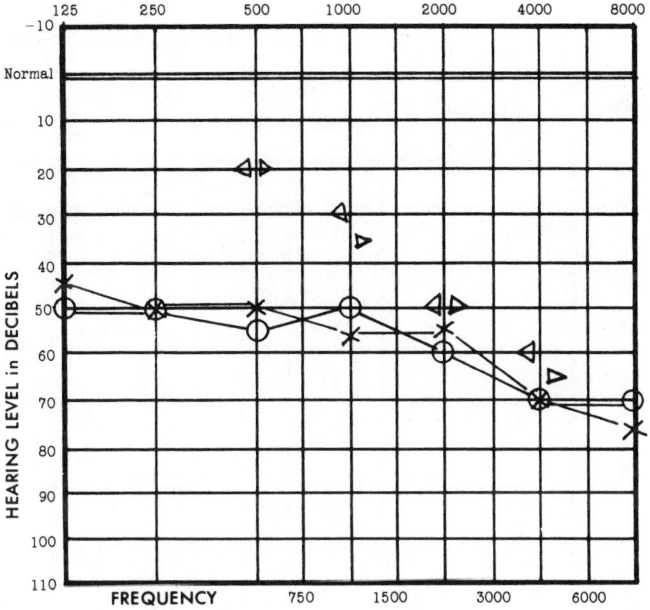

Figure 6.8. AUDIOGRAM

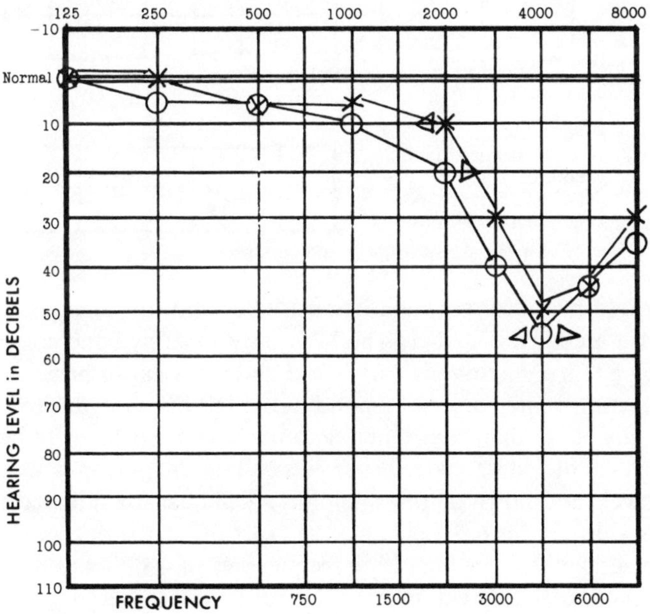

AC = testing by air conduction
BC = testing by bone conduction vibrator

		AC	AC (masked)	BC	BC (masked)
Right	Red*	○	△	>	▷
Left	Blue*	×	□	<	◁

*Color not shown in these audiograms.

Figure 6.9. AUDIOGRAM

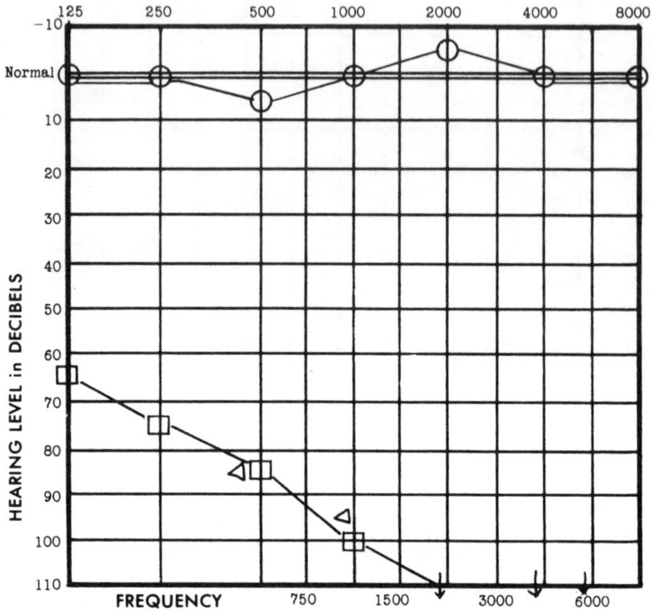

AC = testing by air conduction
BC = testing by bone conduction vibrator

		AC	AC (masked)	BC	BC (masked)
Right	Red*	○	△	>	▷
Left	Blue*	×	□	<	◁

*Color not shown in these audiograms.

threshold levels for air conduction (*O, X*) and for bone conduction (< >) are close together. The high thresholds by bone conduction indicate that something is wrong with the inner ear or nerve. The air conduction scores are correspondingly high because you can never hear any better than your inner ear and nerve are capable of hearing, regardless of testing procedures. Notice that the person whose hearing levels are shown on this audiogram can hear low-pitched sounds quite well, but his hearing begins to taper off at 1,000 Hz and drops quite suddenly at the very high frequencies of 4,000 and 8,000 Hz. This pattern is very common in sensori-neural losses. This hard-of-hearing person hears many of the noises of daily life as well as anyone else, but most of the consonant sounds of speech are lost to him.

The audiogram in Figure 6.7 shows a *mixed impairment,* consisting of a sensori-neural loss plus an additional conductive defect.

Note the spread between the *X* and *O* symbols and the < > symbols. In a purely sensori-neural loss, the symbols for air conduction and bone conduction are close together. In a conductive loss, there is a spread, but the bone conduction results are in the "normal" range. In this case, the bone-conduction results show a loss, and the air-conduction results indicate further loss.

The person whose audiogram is shown in Figure 6.8 has a sensori-neural hearing loss resulting from noise exposure. Note the sharp dip in the 4,000 to 6,000 Hz frequency range. This is a common pattern in noise-induced hearing losses. Unless preventive measures are taken, the hearing impairment is likely to spread to other frequencies.

Figure 6.9 is the audiogram of an individual who has lost most of the hearing in his left ear, while his right ear has remained normal. This is called a *unilateral* impairment (*uni,* "one;" *lateral,* "side"). You will notice by the symbols (□ for air conduction and ◁ for bone conduction) that a masking noise was introduced into the good right ear while the left one was tested, to avoid crossover hearing that would give a false picture of the loss. The arrows pointing downward on the left side of the 2,000, 4,000, and 6,000 Hz lines indicate that the patient gave no response to these tones even at the highest level of loudness available on the audiometer.

When you have your hearing tested, ask for a copy of your audiogram. You can study it at home, with the help of the sample audiograms and explanations in this chapter, to develop a better understanding of the degree and pattern of your loss. Then file it for comparison with future tests of your hearing.

What is my "percentage" of hearing loss? Many people ask this question, but the answer may be misleading. There *is* a formula for calculating percentage of hearing loss, but most audiologists prefer not to use it. The reason is that it fails to take into consideration the *pattern* of the loss, which is of utmost importance in determining a patient's ability to use his hearing for communication. A person with a high-frequency sensori-neural impairment might have a low "percentage" of hearing loss and still have a great amount of difficulty understanding speech. On the other hand, an individual with a flat, conductive pattern may have a high percentage of loss and still hear speech very well with the help of a hearing aid. The best way to estimate the severity of your hearing handicap is to determine your *hearing loss for speech,* which is expressed, not as a percentage, but in decibels.

How is hearing loss for speech calculated? The best and most direct way, of course, is by speech audiometry, as described earlier in this chapter. This test tells how loud speech must be for you to understand it, as well as the amount of difficulty you have in discriminating among the various speech sounds. If speech audiometry is not available to you, it is possible to *estimate* your hearing loss for speech from the results of your pure-tone test.

Can I do this myself? Yes, if you have a copy of your pure-tone audiogram. To estimate the severity of your loss for speech, you need to consider: (1) the amount of loss for the "speech frequencies," and (2) the shape of the curve on your audiogram. Studies have shown that the average of your hearing levels for the frequencies of 500, 1,000, and 2,000 Hz comes close to the hearing loss for speech as measured on a speech audiometer. So, add your decibel levels for these three frequencies. Here's an example from the audiograms we've been studying. In the audiogram in Figure 6.5, the left ear shows a loss of forty-five decibels at 500 Hz, fifty-five decibels at 1,000 Hz, and fifty decibels at 2,000 Hz. So . . .

45 + 55 + 50 = 150 ÷ 3 = 50 decibels
average for left ear.

In the right ear, we have fifty decibels for all three frequencies. Obviously, this person's estimated loss for speech is fifty decibels.

Next, look at your audiogram *curve*. If there is a sudden drop in hearing level between 500 Hz and 1,000 Hz and between 1,000 Hz and 2,000 Hz (twenty decibels or more), you should *omit* the frequency that shows the greatest loss and compute the average of the other two. For example, in the Figure 6.6 audiogram, the hearing level for the left ear at 500 Hz is five decibels, at 1,000 Hz it's thirty decibels, and at 2,000 Hz, fifty decibels. Since the 2,000 Hz reading shows the greatest loss, omit that figure in your computation.

5 + 30 + ~~50~~ = 35 ÷ 2 = 17 decibels
average for left ear.

Right ear, same audiogram:

10 + 35 + ~~55~~ = 45 ÷ 2 = 22 decibels
average for right ear.

If there is *less* than twenty-five decibels difference between the averages of your two ears, the lower figure is the one that represents your hearing loss for speech. In the above example, it is seventeen decibels.

If the averages for left and right ears *differ* by twenty-five decibels or more, add five decibels to the average of the better ear.

Hearing Threshold Level dB (ISO)	Class	Degree of Handicap	Average Hearing Threshold Level for 500, 1000, and 2000 Hz in the Better Ear*		Ability to Understand Speech
			More Than	Not More Than	
	A	Not Significant		25 dB (ISO)	No significant difficulty with faint speech
25	B	Slight Handicap	25 dB (ISO)	40 dB	Difficulty only with faint speech
40	C	Mild Handicap	40 dB	55 dB	Frequent difficulty with normal speech
55	D	Marked Handicap	55 dB	70 dB	Frequent difficulty with loud speech
70	E	Severe Handicap	70 dB	90 dB	Can understand only shouted or amplified speech
90	F	Extreme Handicap	90 dB		Usually cannot understand even amplified speech

Table 6.1. Classes of hearing handicap. From *Hearing and Deafness*, third edition, by Hallowell Davis and S. Richard Silverman. Copyright 1947, 1960, 1970 by Holt, Rinehart & Winston, Inc. Reprinted by permission of Holt, Rinehart & Winston.

Example: If the average threshold for the three frequencies is thirty-seven decibels for the left ear and sixty-two decibels for the right ear, add five decibels to the thirty-seven-decibel figure.

$$37 + 5 = 42 \text{ decibels.}$$

The figure you obtain in this way represents your hearing loss for speech.

Once you've computed these figures, what good are they? They can give you a pretty good idea of the *severity* of your handicap and the *effect* of that handicap on your ability to understand speech.

Locate your level of hearing for speech in Table 6.1, using your score as obtained by speech audiometry or the average you have computed from your pure-tone audiogram. You can see, by looking in the left-hand column, your estimated degree of handicap, and, by consulting the right-hand column, your expected ability to understand speech. Remember that this is only an estimate. Your ability to understand speech is also affected by at least two other factors: your age at the time of onset of loss, and your psychological adjustment.

How does my age at the onset of my loss affect my understanding of speech? If you were born with impaired hearing, or if your loss occurred before you were old enough to develop a solid background in language skills, your handicap for understanding speech is naturally much greater than if you acquired your hearing problem later in life. Hearing is the main channel through which we develop language skills. The child who has a severe hearing loss from birth, or whose impairment occurs during the first year and a half of his life, has to be taught words and the principles of language by a slow, laborious word-by-word process.

A mother once complained to me that there must be something wrong with the way we were handling her teen-age daughter's aural rehabilitation program. The mother had met a young man who was the same age as her daughter and had about the same amount of hearing loss. The young man was in the top third in his class, spoke much more clearly than her daughter, and was a better lipreader. A bit of questioning revealed that the boy had had normal hearing until he developed meningitis at age six. Her daughter was *born* with her hearing impairment. That difference was about as great as the difference between learning to ride a bike normally and learning to do it with an artificial leg. So time of onset is important in *that* way. It may also make some difference at the other end of the age spectrum. Sometimes, by the time we have a sizable number of years tucked away under our belts, we begin to have a bit of difficulty with language, even without a hearing loss. Hardening of the arteries of the brain, a mild stroke, generally poor health, or nervous conditions can cause language problems. Even a mild hearing loss added to these conditions may make speech reception and expression more difficult than would be expected from the hearing loss alone. Yet I can say with complete confidence that no one is too old to benefit from a well-planned and carefully followed program of aural rehabilitation. That's not eyewash. Clinical results with people of all ages prove the truth of it. The person who refuses to try is the only one who can't be helped.

What if I have impaired hearing in only one ear? Naturally, a unilateral hearing impairment is not nearly as handicapping as a bilateral (two-ear) loss. You do have some difficulty in hearing sounds that come from the direction of your "bad" ear, and you have a hard time *locating* sounds and estimating the *distance* from which the sounds originate. This lack of spatial orientation with regard to sound may create some problems for you in group conversation situations. Music may sound "flat" to you. If these problems bother you significantly, you may want to get a hearing aid for your poorer ear, if there is enough usable hearing left in it to make it worth the expense. Your audiologist can tell you whether or not the investment would be worthwhile for you.

What other variable is involved in the degree of handicap a hearing loss causes? A hearing impairment almost always begets some social and psychological adjustment problems for the individual. Our sense of well-being is strongly influenced by our ability to communicate with others. When this ability is hampered, our world seems to shrink. The result can be devastating if we lack the resources for coping with it. In Chapter 12, we'll discuss some of these adjustment problems and offer some very specific suggestions for overcoming them.

We've been talking for several pages about the *handicap* of hearing impairment, so I wouldn't be a bit surprised if, right now, you're feeling a little weighted down by this hearing problem of yours. Maybe the best way to point you upward is to close this chapter with an observation made by John Neal:

"Kites rise against, not with, the wind."

7

Will a hearing aid help me, and if so, how can I choose the right one?

Changing Times magazine reports that "the great majority of the hearing-impaired . . . can be helped through the use of modern-day amplification—by methods that are not complicated, not inconvenient, not unattractive, not uncomfortable and not prohibitively expensive. Yet by a conservative estimate, no more than 25% of the Americans who need help for hearing problems have received it."[1]

If you are among those who could benefit from a hearing aid, but you're struggling along without one, it may be because someone has told you that yours is the kind of loss that can't be helped by an aid. Or maybe you think your loss is not great enough, or that it's too great, or that you're too old to adjust to amplification, or that you can't afford an expensive instrument, or that a hearing aid would call attention to your problem or make you look older than you are. Or maybe you have a hearing aid that didn't do the job for you, or that proved to be too annoying, so you decided you were better off without it.

Most of these reasons were valid a few years ago, but modern technology has recently made some startling advances in hearing aid design, efficiency, and adaptability. As you read this chapter, you may be pleasantly surprised to find that some of your objections to and doubts about what a hearing aid can do for *you* are no longer grounded in fact.

What are these advances? How have hearing aids changed? Any device that helps a person to hear better could be called a hearing aid. The oldest aid to hearing—one that has probably been used as long as man has existed—is the hand cupped behind the ear. This does help somewhat, because it directs more sound waves into the ear, but it is of value only in the slightest degrees of hearing loss. Even in these cases, such maneuvering is far less efficient and certainly more conspicuous than the electrical hearing aid.

Building on this principle of directing more sound waves into the ear, man developed such mechanical aids as ear trumpets, auricles, and speaking tubes. These nonelectrical aids have been used for at least two and a half centuries, and the best of them can make sounds about twenty decibels louder. They still have some limited usefulness for elderly people who resist the idea of "electrical contraptions" or who haven't the patience needed to adjust to more sophisticated means of amplification.

The first electrical hearing aid was made in the United States more than seventy years ago. It was large, awkward, conspicuous, and not very efficient. Great advances followed the invention of the vacuum tube, and when in 1948 the transistor was substituted for the vacuum tube, a minor revolution in hearing aid design took place. Since then, hearing aids have decreased in size and increased in the amount of possible amplification (See Figure 7.1.)

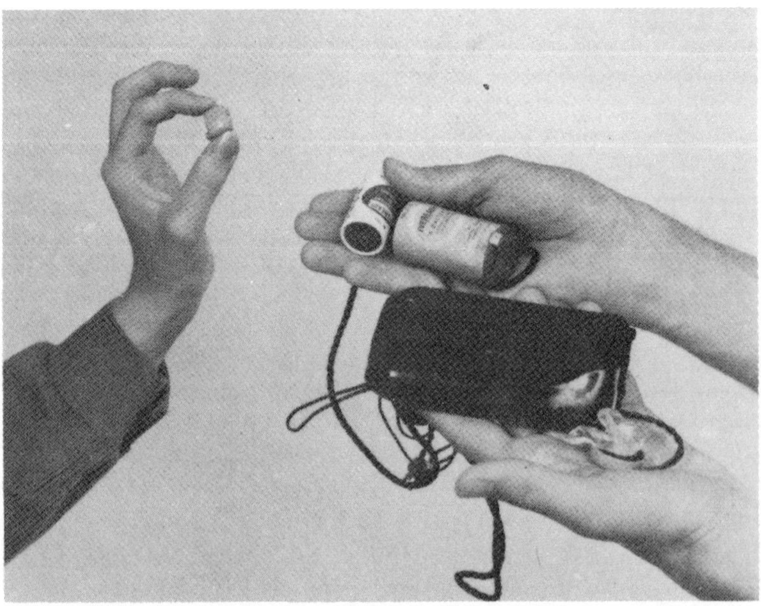

Figure 7.1. *Right,* a body-worn hearing aid of twenty years ago and batteries from an even earlier aid are contrasted with, *left,* a modern, all-in-the-ear model of today.

One problem with the older aids was that, when the volume was turned up enough for the wearer to understand speech, louder sounds (such as banging doors) became painful. It is now possible to *limit the output* of the aid so that it can be set to make *speech* sounds loud enough, while at the same time it keeps *all* sounds below the level of pain for the wearer. This protects him against sudden loud noises, such as a door slamming, a dog barking, or a lawn mower starting up. (See Figure 7.2.)

Another thing that made hearing aid use unpleasant for many people was the fact that, until recently, all frequencies (or pitches) were amplified equally. This worked to the disadvantage of the person with a high-frequency hearing loss. When those higher tones were made loud enough for him to hear them, the lower ones (for which his hearing was normal) became intolerably loud. It is now possible to select a hearing aid with frequency-response characteristics that at least partially compensate for this problem. Further reduction of the low frequencies can be accomplished by modifications made in the individual earmolds.[2] (See Figure 7.3.)

Another advance that has helped make hearing aids suitable for more people is the development of speech audiometry. As I explained in Chapter 6, by a combination of pure-tone testing and speech-audiometric testing, the audiologist or hearing aid dealer can determine a patient's hearing threshold (the level at which he can barely hear a tone or speech sound), his most comfortable loudness level, and his tolerance level (the level at which sounds become uncomfortably loud). All of these measurements help to determine the type of aid and the control settings that will give the wearer the greatest improvement in his hearing without undue distortion and discomfort. Speech audiometry also makes it possible for the hearing aid candidate to compare his scores using various aids, to see which one gives him the best understanding of speech.

Do these advances mean that everyone with a hearing loss can now successfully wear a hearing aid? I wish I could answer yes, but I can't. There are still some people who have out-of-the-ordinary problems and complications that make hearing aid fitting impossible. Still, there's no question that many people who were formerly considered unfittable are now able to benefit from hearing aids. If it's been a few years since you've checked into the possibility of a hearing aid, I'd suggest you do some more investigating.

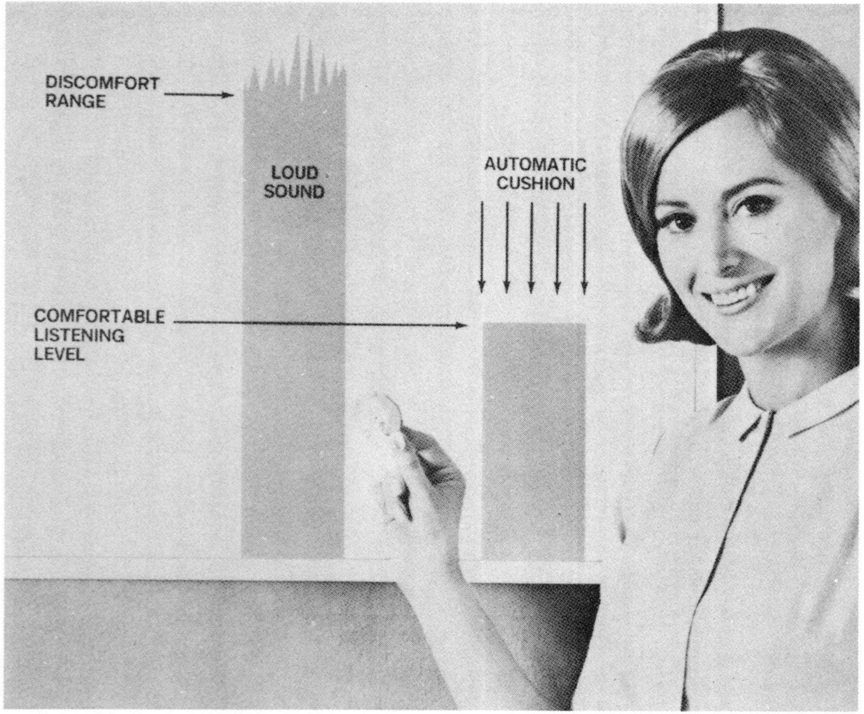

Figure 7.2. Modern hearing aids are set to protect the ear from uncomfortably loud sounds. (Photo courtesy of Zenith Hearing Instrument Corporation, a subsidiary of Zenith Radio Corporation.)

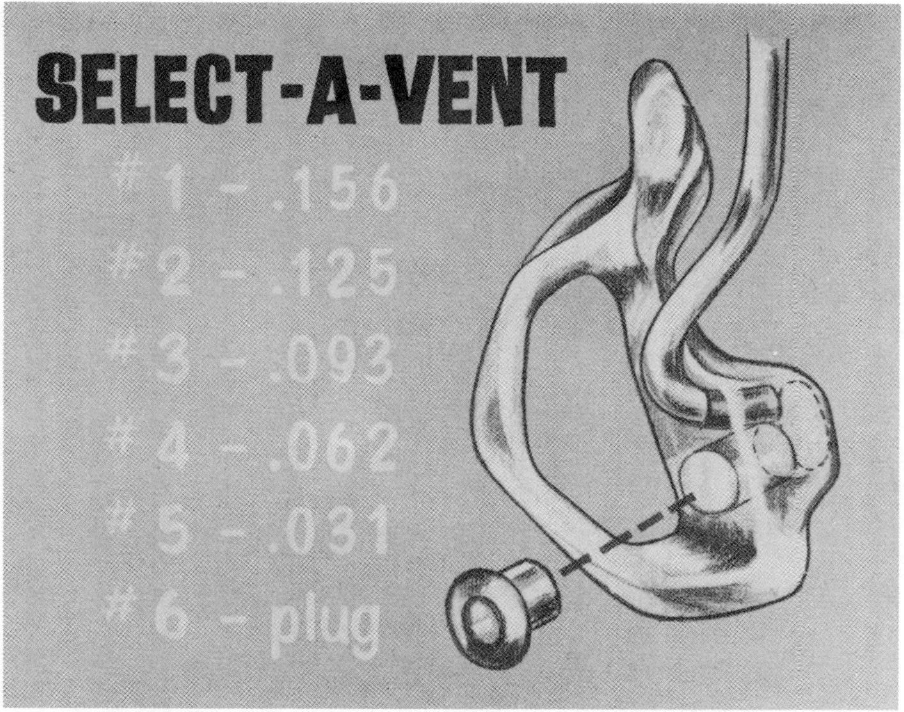

Figure 7.3. This photograph shows one way of modifying an earmold to emphasize the higher frequencies. The numbers represent various sizes of vent opening. (Photo courtesy of Mid States Laboratories, Inc.)

Here are some frequently asked questions. Do any of them fit your situation?

I have only a mild hearing loss. Would a hearing aid help me enough to justify the expense? At one time, it was believed that only those with a loss greater than thirty decibels could benefit from amplification. This is no longer true. As Newby points out:

> The oft-quoted rule that a hearing aid would not be considered unless the hearing loss for speech in the better ear is at least 30 decibels no longer applies, since there are so many exceptions to the "rule." Today's hearing aids are easily put on and taken off. They operate quietly, and many patients with only minimal hearing loss for speech find hearing aids helpful to them, even though they may not be used at all times.[3]

If you have a mild loss, your decision about whether or not to purchase an aid may depend partly on the conditions of your daily life. How important is it for you to be sure of hearing correctly at all times? A judge, for instance, couldn't take a chance on misunderstanding courtroom testimony, and a musician must be sure of hearing without distortion. Do you often have to listen under less-than-ideal conditions? A teacher must be able to hear the students who sit in the back of the classroom, and a student must be able to hear lectures from a distance. Is it important for you to hear weak sounds or quiet speech? An automobile mechanic or TV repairman must be able to detect faint sounds, and a librarian must be able to understand whispered speech. If your hearing loss interferes with communication, or if you feel that you frequently need to strain to hear, then you may want to consider a hearing aid, even if your loss is mild. (Of course, this applies only if medical or surgical correction of your hearing problem has already been ruled out.)

There's another advantage in getting a hearing aid for a mild impairment. *If* you should eventually develop a greater loss, you will have made the adjustment to a hearing aid while adapting is still relatively easy. You will have avoided the "auditory shock" that often comes with learning to hear again when the loss is severe and of long standing.

Would a hearing aid do me any good if I have a loss in only one ear? If your "good" ear is truly unimpaired, you're probably able to hear speech adequately with that ear, no matter how bad the other one is. Still, there are some definite advantages of binaural hearing that you might want to consider. Being able to hear with both ears gives us our ability to tell what direction sounds are coming from and how far away they are. It helps us to follow group conversations as the flow of speech shifts rapidly from one person to another. It makes it easier for us to hear speech against a background of noise, helps us to identify common environmental sounds, reduces listening fatigue, and makes music and other sounds richer and fuller. Many people with unilateral impairments are now being fitted with hearing aids. (See the section later in this chapter on CROS and BICROS hearing aids.)

Will a hearing aid help if I have a conductive hearing loss? As we have seen, conductive hearing losses result from problems in the outer or middle ear. Most people with these losses have "flat" patterns. That is, they hear all frequencies at about the same level of loudness. Newby states that "the person who is likely to benefit most from a hearing aid is one who has a 'flat' conductive loss of 30 to 60 decibels in extent."[4] If your loss is purely conductive, it probably fits in this category. It should be easy for you to get used to a hearing aid because you can tolerate high levels of amplification. This is because your conductive loss protects your inner ear, and also because you don't have the problem of recruitment (rapid buildup of perceived loudness) that the person with a sensori-neural loss has.

It's especially important for you to have a thorough medical evaluation first, though, because there's a good possibility that your problem can be corrected medically or surgically.

What if I don't want to have surgery? It may be that you can choose a hearing aid instead of surgery, but you should consider your decision very carefully. If you have otosclerosis, for instance, you may be a good candidate for *either* a hearing aid or surgery. If you choose the hearing aid route, though, there's always the possibility that the problem in your middle ear could eventually extend into the inner ear. Your age and general health should be taken into consideration, too, in this decision. You may want to get the opinion of more than one medical expert before deciding whether a hearing aid or surgery is the best solution to your problem.

Is it true that hearing aids can't help people who have sensori-neural losses? Let's face it. If you have a high-frequency hearing loss with normal hearing in the lower frequencies, plus a recruitment problem, it will probably be more difficult to fit you with an aid. You'll probably also have more trouble in adjusting to amplification. Still, the forecast isn't as gray as you might think. It just means that more care will be needed in selection and that you will need some very good follow-up help. Hear the encouraging words of H. G. Wallenfels: "Nowadays almost all cases of nerve deafness can be helped with a hearing aid. The question is only, How do I obtain the best instrument for my particular case and what can I expect?"[5] It is possible to select an aid that amplifies the high frequencies more than the low ones. Your own individual earmold can also be modified to *further* reduce the low sounds. The output limiter on your aid can be set so that sudden loud noises are kept below your tolerance level. Obviously, you will need a *very careful and thorough* audiological evaluation by an experienced person who has both pure-tone and speech-audiometric equipment as well as a variety of hearing aids for you to try. Then, you'll need to realize that it's going to take some time and patience for you to get used to your new hearing aid. The step-by-step procedure given in Chapter 8 will help you, and so will your audiologist, who will work closely with you during the adjustment period. Sound like too much bother? The increasing number of satisfied hearing aid users with sensori-neural losses would tell you it's worth the extra effort.

My loss is so severe that I can't understand oral speech, even with a hearing aid. Is there any point in getting one? Let's listen to Akens's answer to that question: "Hearing aids can improve hearing enough so that even the severely deaf can for the first time hear such noises as train whistles, fire engine sirens, and auto horns. They still may be unable to understand speech, but improved hearing improves their safety as well as sense of well being."[6] Just being able to feel the vibrations that speech causes in the aided ear may also alert you to the fact that someone is speaking to you. Then, if you've learned to lip-read, you can turn toward him and pick up visual cues that will help you to understand what he's saying.

Am I too old to adjust to a hearing aid? This is not an easy question to answer. Who is old, anyway? Where do we draw the line between middle age and old age? I know an eighty-five-year-old lady who is much "younger," mentally and physically, than another friend of mine who is seventy-five.

Several factors should enter into your decision about a hearing aid. For instance, is your eyesight adequate? Vision is a great help in understanding speech if your hearing is poor. If you can see reasonably well, hearing aid adjustment will be easier for you. How's your general health? If you suffer from chronic pain, or if you're unusually weak or highly nervous, getting used to a hearing aid may be just too much of a strain for you. Is there an understanding family member who will help and encourage you while you're adapting to the aid? Silverman and Davis make this recommendation: "When there appears to be any possibility of benefit, we strongly suggest a trial period with the hearing aid during which the person is encouraged but not forced to use the instrument. If he himself then expresses a desire to have the hearing aid, it should be purchased."[7] (We'll talk more about trial periods for hearing aids later in this chapter.)

The Veterans Administration reports having a high degree of success with elderly users of hearing aids. Wallenfels conducted a review of fifty cases of nerve deafness in people between the ages of sixty-five and ninety. He found that, two to three years after the original evaluation, thirty-eight of the fifty were wearing their original instruments, successfully. Three others failed to adjust, two showed inconclusive results, and seven were "unfittable."[8]

In addition to the situations I've described so far, there's another reason why some poeple object to wearing a hearing aid. Let's talk about that fragile thing called vanity.

Won't a hearing aid just call attention to itself and make my problem more obvious? Most modern hearing aids are quite inconspicuous and blend in with a person's appearance better than eyeglasses do. The person whose hearing loss is really conspicuous is the one who says, "What?" or "Huh?" all the time, often misunderstands, and has a straining-to-hear look on his face. If a hearing aid can keep you from doing these things, it will make your problem *less* noticeable instead of *more* obvious. Silverman and Davis have this to say about the man or woman whose hearing is failing: "His friends will welcome his use of a hearing aid because it spares them the painful necessity of having to shout and repeat for him. In fact, *it shows lack of consideration for his family and friends when the hard-of-hearing person does not wear a hearing aid if he can possibly do so and benefit by it.*"[9]

Doesn't a hearing aid make a person "look old"? Did you know that the same complaint used to be made about eyeglasses? When I was a youngster, kids with glasses were called "four eyes," but when my mother was a child, wearing glasses brought shouts of "granny!"

Now, people of *all* ages wear glasses without any stigma at all, and the same kind of acceptance of hearing aids is not far behind. An article in *Changing Times* states: "Nowadays the fear that a hearing aid makes you 'look old' is disappearing rapidly. Young veterans wear hearing aids like Purple Hearts, and youngsters show off their aids, available in bright colors instead of neutral hues."[10]

O K. So you've decided you might give a hearing aid a chance to help you. Now you want to know more about these little "mechanical marvels." Are these the questions you're asking?

How does a hearing aid work? An electrical hearing aid can be compared to a telephone, because both instruments take sound waves and change them into electrical signals and then back into sound waves

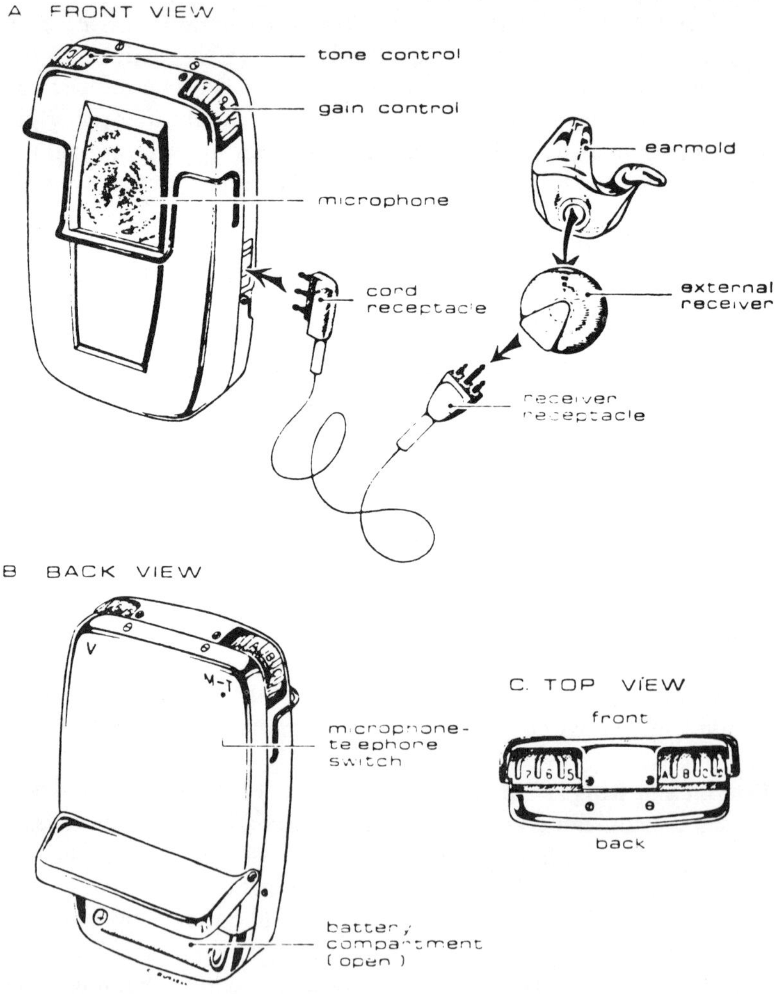

Figure 7.4. Typical body-type aid. (From Alfred L. Miller and Roger Lehman, *A Practical Guide on Hearing Impaired Children,* 1970. Courtesy of Charles C. Thomas, Publisher, Springfield, Illinois.)

again. First, the *microphone* of your hearing aid picks up the sounds around you and converts these into electrical impulses. Then, the *amplifier* in your hearing aid increases the strength of the signals. Finally, the *receiver* changes these amplified electrical signals back into sound waves again. A specially fitted *earmold* fits snugly in your ear and connects the receiver with your ear canal. A *battery* provides the energy for this whole operation. Figures 7.4, 7.5, and 7.6, show you where the various parts are located on different types of hearing aids.

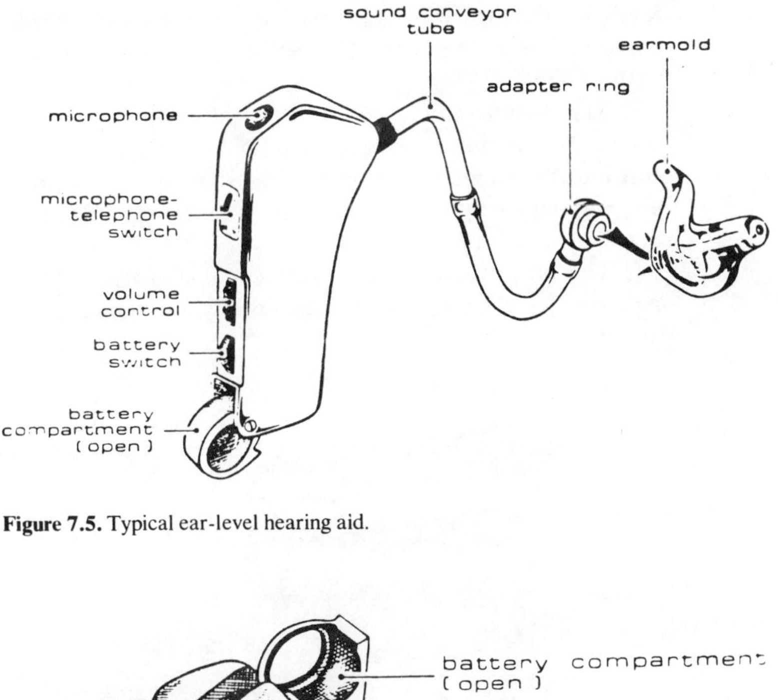

Figure 7.5. Typical ear-level hearing aid.

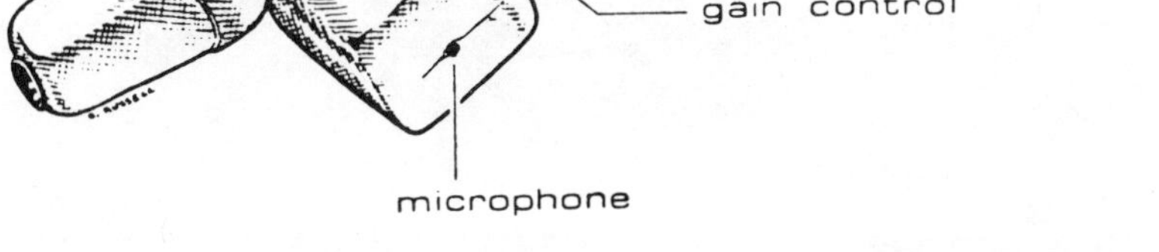

Figure 7.6. Typical in-the-ear hearing aid. (Figs. 7.5 and 7.6 from Alfred L. Miller and Roger Lehman, *A Practical Guide on Hearing Impaired Children,* 1970. Courtesy of Charles C. Thomas, Publisher, Springfield, Illinois.)

What are the different styles of wearable hearing aids? There are four basic types:

1. The body-worn aid has a case about half the size of your shirt pocket. The case, which holds the microphone, amplifier, and batteries, can be carried in your pocket or attached to your clothing. A cord connects this part with the receiver and earmold in your ear. See Figure 7.7.
2. The behind-the-ear aid is smaller, and its microphone, amplifier, battery, and receiver are all in one unit that fits snugly behind the ear. A short plastic tube carries the amplified sound into the earmold. (See Figures 7.8, 7.9, and 7.10.)
3. The eyeglass type of hearing aid is similar to the behind-the-ear model except that the electrical parts are built into the frame of a pair of glasses. A tiny transparent tube with an eartip brings the sound into the ear. (See Figures 7.11 and 7.12.)
4. The all-in-the-ear aid is very small and light. As its name implies, the whole thing fits directly into the ear, with part of it extending into the ear canal. (See Figure 7.13.)

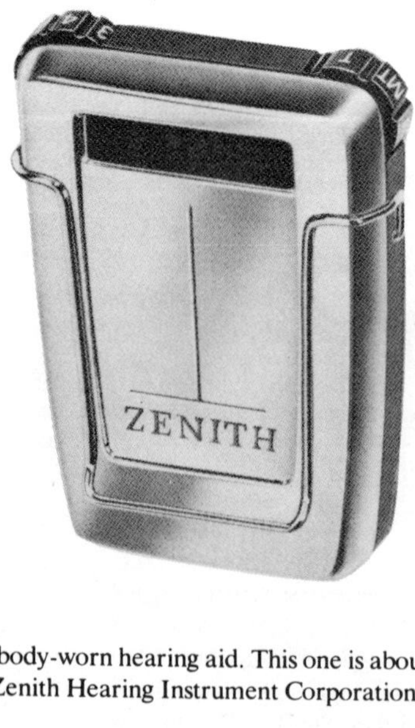

Figure 7.7. A typical body-worn hearing aid. This one is about the size of a cigarette lighter. (Courtesy of Zenith Hearing Instrument Corporation, a subsidiary of Zenith Radio Corporation.)

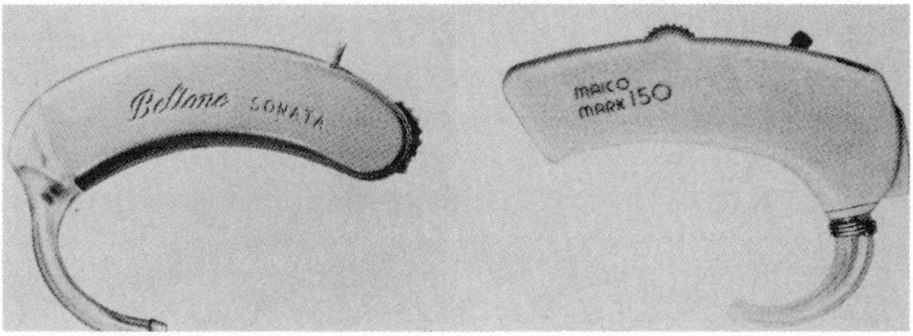

Figures 7.8 and 7.9. Two typical behind-the-ear hearing aids, differing somewhat in size and placement of controls. (Fig. 7.8 courtesy of Beltone Electronics Corporation. Fig. 7.9 courtesy of Maico Hearing Instruments.)

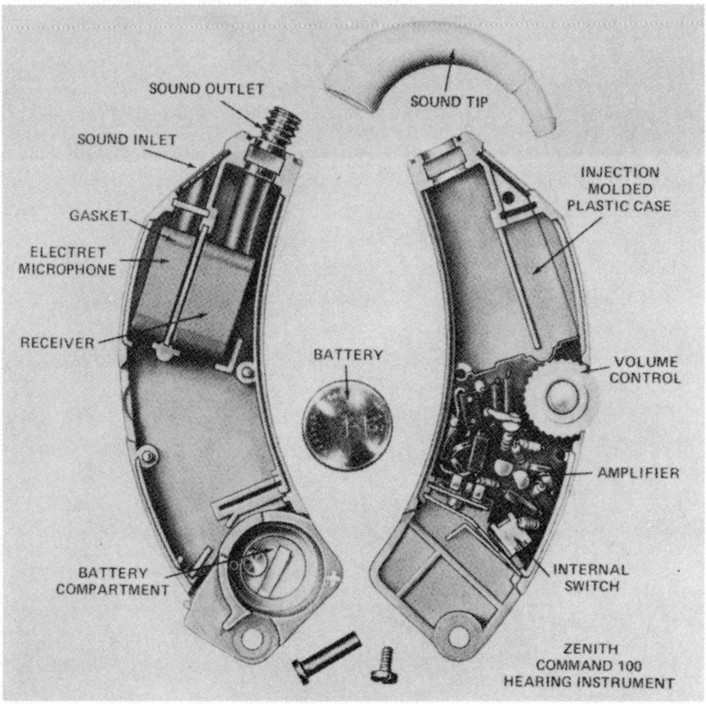

Figure 7.10. This photograph shows the inner mechanism of the Command 100 behind-the-ear aid. (Courtesy of Zenith Hearing Instrument Corporation, a subsidiary of Zenith Radio Corporation.)

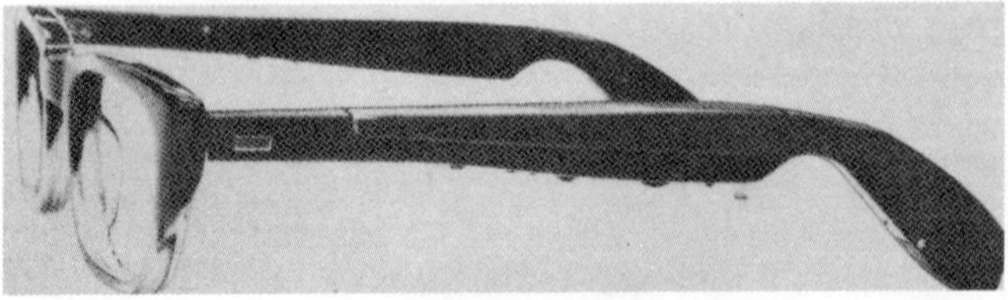

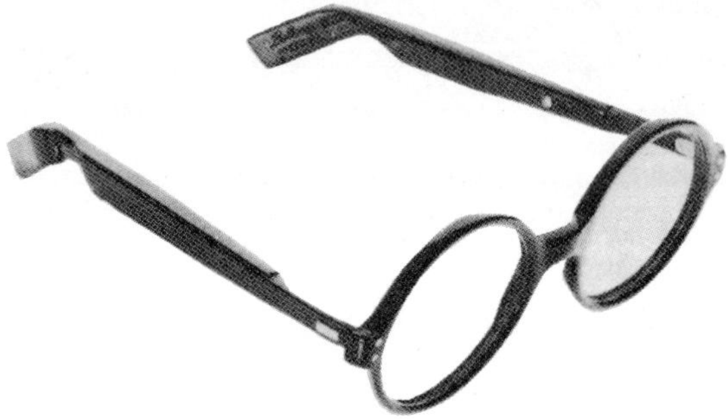

Figures 7.11 and 7.12. Here are two different styles of eyeglass hearing aids. (Fig. 7.11 courtesy of Maico Hearing Instruments. Fig. 7.12 courtesy of Beltone Electronics Corporation.)

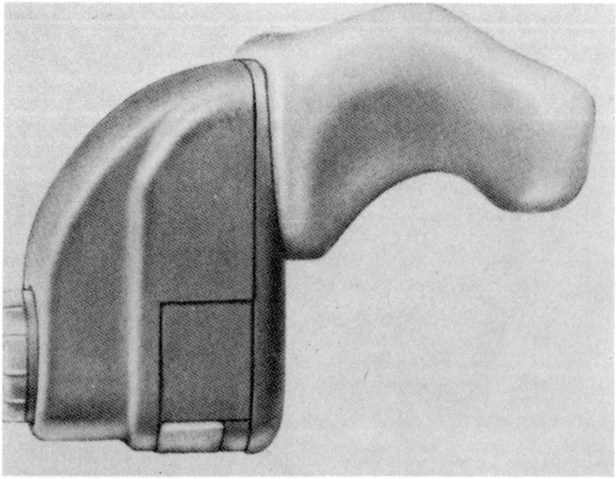

Figure 7.13. A typical in-the-ear aid, weighing less than battery. Projection on the right side is the canal earmold Electronics Corporation.)

How can I tell which is the best aid for me? There is no single hearing aid that's suitable for all types of hearing loss. Of course, price and appearance are important to you, but you should not base your choice of a hearing aid on these factors alone. It's much more important for you to select the hearing aid that will do the most for you in terms of improving your hearing ability. A tiny hearing aid that is inconspicuous will be of little value to you if it doesn't amplify sound enough for your particular hearing loss. If you have a severe or profound loss, you'll probably need a body-worn aid. Behind-the-ear and eyeglass aids are generally suitable for people with mild to moderate losses. If your hearing loss is mild, and if you don't need special frequency emphasis, an in-the-ear model may be what you need.

What does the earmold do? The purpose of the earmold is to seal in the amplified sound. Ear canals are like fingerprints. No two are alike, so your hearing aid dealer or audiologist will make an impression of your ear canal. This impression will be sent to a laboratory that specializes in making custom earmolds, so that yours will fit your ear comfortably and provide the best results. Figures 7.14, 7.15, and 7.16 are representative of various types of earmolds. If you have a high frequency loss, your earmold can be modified in ways that keep the low frequency sounds from becoming too loud for you. This may be done by changing the length of the part of the earmold that fits in your ear canal, or by making an opening in the earmold. The latter process is called *venting*.

What brand of hearing aid is best? There are close to a hundred different brands of hearing aids. Brand name is important, of course, because it tells you who is responsible for the technical workings of a very complicated mechanism. You'll also want to consider such things as availability of service, the dealer's experience, and his reputation for working with his clients after the sale. Wallenfels points out that "in these days of rapid travel, it is of real value to a hearing aid wearer to operate an instrument which carries the name of a well-known manufacturer who guarantees nation-wide, perhaps even world-wide, service."[11]

If possible, you should consult an audiologist who does not sell hearing aids but who has a variety of brands and models for you to try out. Many colleges and universities offer degrees in speech pathology and audiology and can give you very good hearing aid evaluations in their clinics. For information about qualified audiologists in your area, write to American Speech-Language-Hearing Association, 10801 Rockville Pike, Rockville, MD 20852.

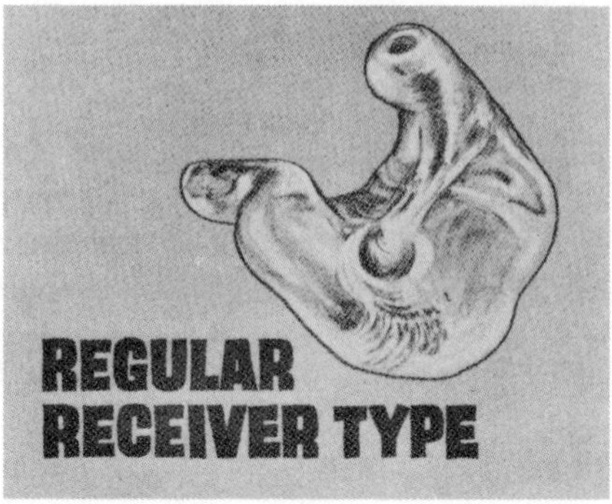

Figure 7.14. Regular earmold, designed for body-worn aids that have the receiver at the ear. (Figs. 7.14, 7.15, and 7.16 courtesy of Mid States Laboratories, Inc.)

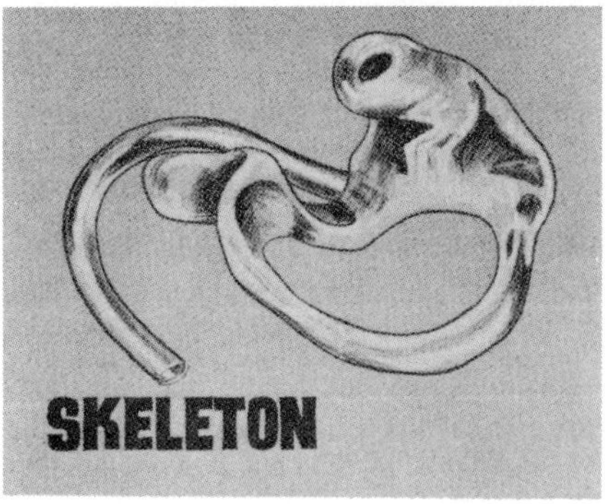

Figure 7.15. Skeleton earmold, for use with head-worn aids. It has a minimum frame with a hollow center for lightness, firm retention, and excellent concealment.

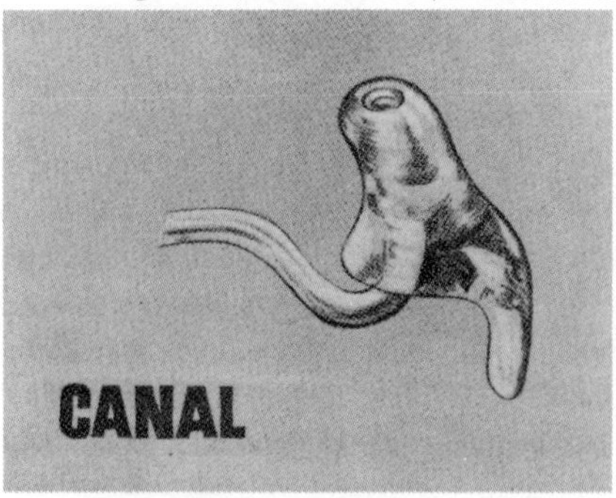

Figure 7.16. Canal earmold. Primarily built for use with head-worn instruments. Offers excellent concealment as it is actually worn within the ear canal. Recommended for mild losses only.

To locate a speech and hearing center near you, write to the above address or to the National Association for Hearing and Speech Action, 814 Thayer Avenue, Silver Spring, MD 20910.

A free booklet is available on results of government comparative testing of brand-name hearing aids. It is, *Hearing Aids,* Catalog No. 312C, available from Consumer Information, Public Documents Distribution Center, Pueblo, CO, 81009.

The Veterans Administration also publishes a booklet every year, entitled *Hearing Aids Selected*. Some manufacturers choose not to submit their products for VA evaluation, though, so if you order this booklet, remember that not all brands are included. Write to Veterans Administration Supply Service, Department of Medicine and Surgery, Washington, DC 20420.

One word of caution. An aid that was judged to be effective for one person may not work for you at all, and the reverse is also true.

How can I judge the reliability of a hearing-aid dealer? A pamphlet put out by the Better Business Bureau says that:

> The answers to the following questions may help you to evaluate your hearing aid dealer:
>
> How long has the dealer been in business?
>
> Does he have an established office?
>
> Is he a member of the National Hearing Aid Society?
>
> Is he a member of the State or City Hearing Aid Dealers Guild or Society?
>
> If your state licenses hearing aid dealers, does he hold such a license?
>
> Does he stand behind his product and clearly spell out his warranty or guarantee?
>
> Does he represent and promote his products openly and honestly?
>
> Can he provide rapid and efficient repairs if your hearing aid needs to be serviced?
>
> If in doubt about the reputation of a hearing aid dealer, investigate before you purchase by calling your Better Business Bureau.[12]

Whatever you do, don't order a hearing aid out of a catalog, no matter how appealing the price may be. Such aids are mass-produced and, though the quality *may* be adequate, it is essential for you to have an individual evaluation of your particular type and degree of loss as well as personal follow-up help in adjusting to your aid. Neither of these can be supplied by mail! For information about qualified hearing aid dealers in your area, write to National Hearing Aid Society, 20361 Middlebelt Road, Livonia, MI 48152.

Should I have amplification for both ears or just one? The experts can't agree on the answer to this one. Sanders asserts that "hearing-aid users who have switched from the use of monaural (one-ear) to binaural (two-ear) aids frequently list, among the improvements that they notice, such factors as better comprehension of speech in noisy situations, greater ability to follow conversational speech in group situations, better hearing of speech at a distance, and more natural sound reproduction."[13] On the other hand, Jerger, Carhart, and Dirks report that "there remains little concrete evidence that binaural amplification actually produces any significant improvement in the ability to understand speech."[14]

If, after a careful evaluation of your hearing in both ears, your audiologist recommends binaural amplification, you may want to work out a trial plan with the dealer. Binaural amplification is easy to achieve with eyeglass aids or behind-the-ear models. If your hearing loss is about the same in both ears, you may want to consider a Y-cord aid. This is a body-worn instrument using a single amplifying system with a receiver in each ear. It's less expensive than a system with two separate units, but it won't work for you if there's a significant difference between your ears.

You should definitely *not* use amplification in both ears if the "tone" of the hearing aid is worse when the second ear is added, or if the addition of the second aid makes sounds uncomfortably loud for you, or if your understanding of speech is better with one aid than it is with two.

If I have only one hearing aid, which ear should be fitted? Your audiologist or hearing aid dealer will know which is best. If your better ear has enough hearing left to be of some use *without* an aid, he'll probably fit the poorer ear. This way, your hearing level in the two ears will be more nearly balanced. On the other hand, if your hearing impairment is severe or profound, he's more likely to fit the better ear since your poorer ear, even with an aid, might not be of much help. In this case, the object is to provide the best improvement possible on the ear that has the greater potential. There are exceptions to these guides, though, and other factors that must be considered, so accept the decision of the expert who works with you.

What are *CROS* and *BICROS* hearing aids? A major breakthrough, that's what. These recently developed aids are helping many people who were once considered unfittable. If you have a unilateral loss, or if your loss is in both ears, but there's a steep drop-off in the high frequencies, maybe this unique system has possibilities for you.

In 1965, Harford and Barry of Northwestern University reported success in what they called contralateral routing of signals, or CROS.[15] With this system, the microphone is placed on the side of the poorer ear and the sound is transferred to a receiver in the better ear. A special earmold leaves the "good" ear open to pick up sounds unaided, at the same time that it receives amplified sounds coming from the other side. It is easy to see how this could help the person with one "good" and one "bad" ear. But, surprisingly, this system also makes if possible to successfully fit another group of people who had previously had poor results with hearing aids. These are individuals who have normal or near normal hearing for the low frequencies and a sharp drop-off for the higher tones. They are the "I-hear-you-but-I can't-understand-you" people. Conventional hearing aids usually "drive these people out of their gourds," to quote my husband's terminology. This is because, until the CROS came along, there was no really satisfactory way to make the high frequencies loud enough without also increasing the low frequencies to an uncomfortably loud level. The open earpiece in the CROS aid *suppresses* the low frequencies while it allows the high ones to be greatly amplified. If there is quite a bit of difference in the hearing patterns of your two ears, two microphones are used, but the sound is still fed into the better ear. This two-microphone system is called the BICROS. CROS and BICROS aids are available in either behind-the-ear models mounted on a headband or in eyeglass-type models. (See Figures 7.18 and 7.19.)

Alfred Dunlavy believes that the CROS fitting will almost double the number of people who can benefit from the use of hearing aids.[16] That's exciting news! Could this be the breakthrough *you've* been praying for?

How do the controls on a hearing aid work? All hearing aids have a volume control, sometimes called the *gain control*. This adjusts the intensity of the signal your ear receives. The *tone control* allows you to increase or decrease the relative amplification of the high, middle, or low frequencies. The *output limiter* makes it possible to limit the level of loudness so that amplified sound is never permitted to exceed your tolerance level. When your aid is turned up enough to make speech understandable, the output limiter protects you from the "auditory shock" of sudden loud noises, such as banging doors. Your audiologist or hearing aid dealer will know where this control should be set for your individual hearing tolerance level.

How much will a hearing aid cost? If you haven't priced them, you

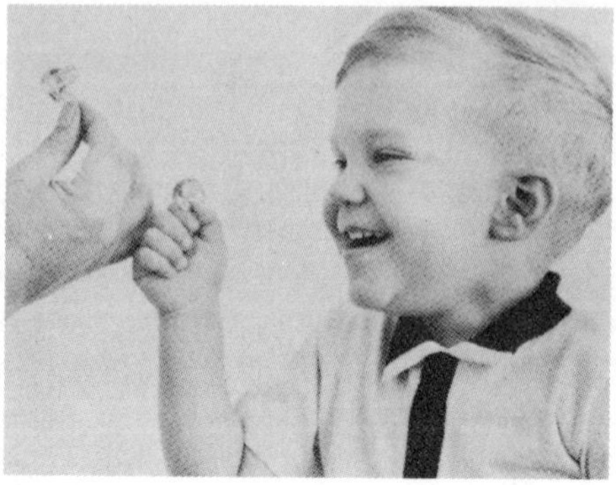

Figure 7.17. shows the size of a regular-type earmold. (Courtesy of Zenith Hearing Instrument Corporation, a subsidiary of Zenith Radio Corporation.)

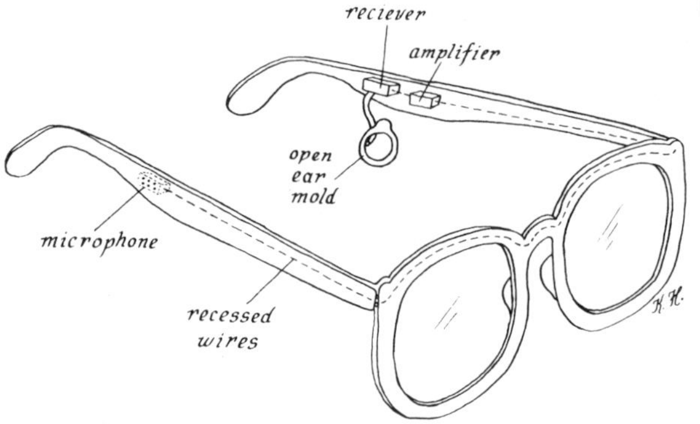

Figure 7.18. A CROS hearing aid, which picks up sound on the side of the poorer ear and delivers it to the better ear.

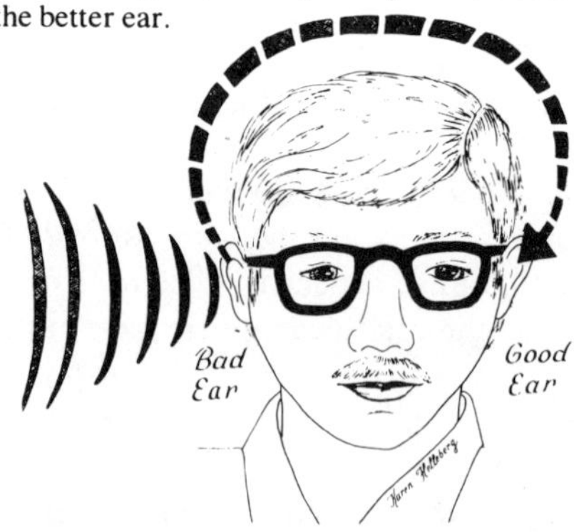

Figure 7.19. A CROS hearing aid transfers sound from a microphone on the side of the "bad" ear to a receiver on the side of the "good" ear. This is done through wires running through eyeglasses, or, in some instances, through a band connecting behind-the-ear aids.

may need your smelling salts. In 1977, the price range for one-ear aids was from below $100 to about $450. Binaural, or two-ear systems, were about double that amount. The price may include the cost of the earmold, rental fees during a trial period, service during the guarantee period, and continuing assistance throughout the life of the aid. Do not shop around for the cheapest aid you can find. An inexpensive instrument of poor quality will be of little use to you if it doesn't deliver the amount of amplification you need or if it continually needs to be repaired. On the other hand, don't assume that the highest priced one is best just because it costs more. You may find satisfaction with one that is moderately priced.

Can I try out an aid before I commit myself to buying it? At the time of this writing, the U.S. Federal Trade Commission is holding hearings on a proposal that would give buyers a thirty-day trial period, after which they could return their hearing aid and get most of their money back. Many dealers are already offering such trials. A rental fee is sometimes charged, but usually this can be applied toward the purchase price of the aid. A pamphlet put out by the Better Business Bureau recommends that you insist on a trial period. "This period can range from two weeks to several months. This will give you an opportunity to use the aid under different conditions. Within a few weeks you should know whether or not the aid is working adequately for you."[17]

If you're trying out a hearing aid, don't be too quick about rejecting it. Remember that you've been hearing in a distorted or weakened way for quite a while. In a sense, you'll have to get used to hearing again, and this may be a little nerve jangling at first. And don't expect miracles. You probably won't hear "perfectly," even with a hearing aid. If you expect too much, you're almost sure to be disappointed. Read Chapter 8 before trying out an aid.

Are there some guidelines I can follow in comparing various aids? Yes. Here are some that may help you.

1. Ask a friend to read a passage from a book or magazine while you wear first one aid and then another. See which one seems to give you the greater ability to *understand* speech.

2. Listen for internal noise. Some aids have more electrical noise than others.

3. In deciding which aid has the best sound *quality,* lean toward the *crisp* rather than the *mellow,* even if it sounds somewhat unnatural to you. Remember that the sound you're *used to hearing* is distorted.

4. Try each aid in a noisy situation. Remember that adjustment will be tough in such conditions, even with the best aid. Your purpose, at this point, is to decide which aid produces the *least* amount of difficulty for you in such situations.

Can I get a free hearing aid, or financial help in buying one? If you need a hearing aid but can't afford one, financial assistance is available through several channels. If you're eligible for Medicaid, you should check to see whether your state's Medicaid program offers assistance.

If you are a veteran, you can receive, at no charge, a complete medical examination of your ears and a professional audiological evaluation at one of the forty-five VA hearing centers around the country, and possibly a free hearing aid. Contact your nearest VA hospital or regional office. Transportation to the nearest VA hearing center will be paid.[18]

If you can't get financial assistance through your state Medicaid or the VA, your local physician, dealer, or a speech and hearing center may be able to refer you to an agency that can help you. Or you can write or call your local United Fund or other social service organization or your state vocational rehabilitation or public health department.

Can a hearing aid do more than help me to hear better? Sounds like kind of a ridiculous question, but the answer is yes. When you begin to hear better, your speech will improve; your relationships with your family should be smoother (no more arguments about TV volume, no more need to shout, no more misunderstandings and hurt feelings); you will probably become more confident on the job; and you'll feel more like socializing and seeking new experiences. This is not to say that a hearing aid will solve all of your problems. But, if your audiologist feels you can benefit from amplification, an aid should make many of those problems easier to face.

Bill Cosby told a joke on the "Johnny Carson Show" the other night that you may appreciate after reading this *long* chapter.

> COSBY: I had a terrible hearing loss and I went all over the world looking for a hearing aid that would help. Finally, my doctor sent me to Japan, where I was fitted with a marvelous hearing aid. I can hear perfectly now.
>
> CARSON: What kind is it?
>
> COSBY: Oh, about 11:45.[19]

Part Two

What can I do to overcome my hearing loss?

8

How can I learn to use my hearing aid successfully?

"What a waste of money *this* contraption is! Worst investment I ever made!" Charles H., a tall, distinguished-looking businessman whose wavy hair was beginning to gray at the temples, walked into my office one day with his hearing aid in his hand and plunked it down on my desk.

"How long have you had the aid?" I asked.

"Oh, couple-three weeks I guess. Wore it to the store the day after I got it and about went crazy. Came home with a splitting headache. I bought it so I could function better in my business, but this nerve-jangling thing's worse than not hearing!"

Mr. H.'s experience is not at all unusual. The disappointment and frustration so many people experience with a new hearing aid is similar to what my seven-year-old son felt when he got a bike for his birthday. He expected to jump on and ride right off, but he found out that it just doesn't work that way.

It's only fair to tell you, *before* you buy a hearing aid, that you're going to have to pedal uphill for a while. You'll have to learn to hear again, and that's not easy. Neither is going to the dentist nor adjusting to contact lenses, but the rewards are worth the effort.

Why is a new hearing aid so irritating? Long before you noticed that you were hard of hearing, before you started having difficulty understanding speech, you had already lost the ability to hear such sounds as those of your own clothing, the squeaking of a chair, the humming of a fluorescent light, a dripping faucet, the rustling of a newspaper. You had grown used to a softening of such loud sounds as a door slamming, a horn honking, and the dog barking. Your new hearing aid causes all of these sounds, which you haven't really heard for years, to invade your noise-cushioned world. It's a little like having someone suddenly shine a spotlight in your eyes when you've been sitting in a dimly lighted room. The shock makes you cringe. Later on in this chapter, we'll give you some step-by-step procedures for overcoming this "auditory shock."

But there must be something wrong with my hearing aid. It has such a peculiar sound to it. Why does everything sound so unnatural? The chances are that what you've been hearing without the aid is unnatural. For instance, without the aid you may have been hearing the lower-pitched sounds but not the higher frequencies; so what you heard was actually distorted. If your hearing aid has been properly fitted to your loss, it compensates for this, at least to some extent, so the tone of what you hear is different. That's why it sounds strange to you at first.

How can I be hard of hearing and yet be so painfully sensitive to noise? It *does* seem odd that many people with hearing losses are unusually touchy about noise, but it's just one of the characteristics of sensori-neural loss. As I explained in Chapter 4, this is called recruitment, and it means that there's an abnormally rapid build-up of the sensation of loudness. As soon as sounds become loud enough to be heard, just a little more increase in loudness brings pain. That's why certain levels of loudness hurt your ears, even though people with normal hearing are perfectly comfortable with the same sounds. This causes some problems in hearing aid fitting. Your audiologist can measure this recruitment factor, so that your hearing aid can be adjusted to keep all sounds *below* your threshold of pain. However, studies have shown that your level of tolerance can be increased to give you a wider range of usable hearing, and this is one of the goals of auditory training. (See Chapter 10.)

Then there's another element that enters into this idea of "noise." What is noise, anyway? Maybe I can make my point best by telling you about an incident that happened in our family. A few months after the astronauts landed on the moon, my mother came to visit us. There was a gem show in town, and my husband asked my mother if she would like to take the children to the rock show. "I think you'd enjoy it," he said. "The moon rocks will be there."

My mother threw up her hands and said, "No *thanks!* I don't care *who's* playing. That kind of music hurts my ears!"

The point is that our reactions are often based on preconceived ideas of what we like or dislike. What's noise to one person may be music to another, so one definition of noise could be "any unwanted sound." For a while after you get your hearing aid, you'll be annoyed by quite a few unwanted sounds. You'll eventually get to feel comfortable with many of them, but there will always be some unwanted sounds in your life, whether you wear a hearing aid or have normal hearing. (Just don't blame your hearing aid for Alice Cooper!)

Will I hear perfectly once I get used to the aid? Unfortunately, a hearing aid is not a substitute ear. This tool for hearing that man has designed is an amazing piece of equipment, but it doesn't compare with the marvelous mechanism God designed—the human ear. For example, an ear with a sensori-neural loss may be unable to hear high tones, no matter how much they're amplified. If all the nerve fibers that normally react to these high frequencies are dead, then no hearing aid could possibly make these tones audible. Happily, even people with very severe losses generally still have some usable hearing left, but it may be limited to just certain frequencies. In these cases, a hearing aid may make speech intelligible, even though the sound of it is still distorted. But isn't that better than not being able to understand at all? Even people with normal hearing get used to putting up with some distortion when they talk on the phone or listen to the radio. The telephone actually cuts out some of the frequencies and distorts others, in the same way that a hearing loss does. But the partial pattern it does transmit is enough to make understanding possible. That's all we need ask of a good hearing aid.

Can a hearing aid make speech intelligible for every wearer? No. Sometimes the loss is so great that even the most powerful hearing aid does not make speech sounds distinguishable for the wearer. In such cases, a hearing aid may still be advisable, for two reasons. First, even though the wearer can't understand speech with his aid, the device may make him aware of noises that could signal danger for him—for example, the honking of a car horn, a shout or a scream, a fire alarm siren. Second, just the vibrations the sound waves cause in his hearing aid may alert the deaf person to the fact that someone is talking. Then he can turn toward the speaker and visually read his speech.

There is also an in-between degree of loss, for which a hearing aid makes speech audible enough that the wearer can catch enough key words to follow a conversation with the help of lipreading, even though he doesn't hear every word.

Will an aid help to restore some of the hearing I have lost? Occasionally an overly enthusiastic salesman leads a client to believe that this will happen, but it is a false claim. You could wear your hearing aid every day for years, but your hearing without the aid would continue to be defective (unless, of course, surgery or other medical techniques are also employed. See Chapter 5).

Can a hearing aid damage the hearing I have left? No. A hearing aid neither injures nor cures an abnormal ear. It's true that, once you get used to hearing better by wearing the aid, you'll notice your loss more when you don't have it on. This is not an indication that your hearing is getting worse, but a sign that you are beginning to take better hearing for granted. That's good.

But my hearing really *could* get worse, couldn't it? If you have a progressive type of loss, it could get worse, but this has nothing to do with your hearing aid. Still, it points up the importance of follow-up testing. You should definitely see your otologist and audiologist at least once a year—more frequently if they request it.

Must I do this even if I have a nerve loss that's not medically correctable? Yes. The audiologist will want to know whether or not your loss is becoming greater, so that he can plan for the right kinds of rehabilitation. Also, it sometimes happens that a person with a sensorineural loss develops problems in the outer and/or middle ear on top of it. This is one thing you don't need! If you see your otologist periodically, he will have a chance to catch this sort of thing early, while it's still likely to be correctable.

Here's a note on the positive side: Like eyesight, hearing often drops to a certain degree of loss and then levels off, never getting much worse. But how can you know whether or not the thief is still in the house unless you call in the authorities?

How long will it take me to adjust to my aid? That's like asking how long it will take to learn to ride a bike. In both cases, the answer depends a lot on the personality of the learner, his motivation, the amount of self-confidence he has, how often he practices, and his age. There are at least two other factors that affect the amount of time it will take you to adjust to your aid: The length of time you have had poor hearing and the *type* of hearing loss you have.

How does duration of loss influence adjustment? Generally, the longer you have been hard of hearing, the longer it will take you to get used to those sounds you have missed for so long, and to relearn to distinguish the various speech sounds. You'll have a lot of catching up to do! This is part of the reason why early detection is so vital.

Why do people with one type of loss adapt to a hearing aid more easily than those with another type? Most people who have a "flat" conductive hearing defect experience very little difficulty in getting used to a hearing aid. In this type of loss, the inner ear and the nerve pathway to the brain are normal, but some problem in the middle or outer ear obstructs the free flow of sound waves to the inner ear. The sound could be heard perfectly if it could get through. Such an individual usually hears all frequencies, or pitches, at about the same level of loudness, so his audiogram pattern is relatively flat. People whose conductive losses cannot be medically or surgically corrected are excellent candidates for hearing aids, because all they need is more loudness to get the signal through, and there is no problem with distortion.

On the other hand, a person with a *sensori-neural* loss is likely to have a much greater loss in some frequencies (usually the higher ones) than in others. So a hearing aid that makes the *high* tones loud enough for him to hear may make the low ones much *too* loud. Modern hearing aids can compensate for this effect to some degree, but not completely, so speech sounds continue to be distorted for this wearer. He is also likely to have a problem with 'recruitment' (low tolerance for loudness), which will limit the amount of amplification he can accept, while the person with a conductive loss can tolerate as much loudness as his loss requires.

Whichever type of loss you have, it is very important for you to find out, from the audiologist, just how much hearing ability you may expect to have with your aid, what you may *not* be able to hear, and how much distortion you should be prepared to put up with. Only by discovering what the hearing aid *cannot* do for you can you ever be satisfied with the results.

Now that I understand some of the problems that confront new hearing aid wearers, how can I overcome them? When you first get your hearing aid, do *not* try to use it in social situations. Do not wear it away from home until you have made a reasonably good adjustment to it at home. Practice the steps that follow, in the order they are given.[1]

The first thing you'll need to do is to get reaccustomed to living with the nonspeech sounds that are a part of daily living. If possible, try to arrange to be alone in the house for a few hours each day, for the first few days or weeks. During this alone time, sit down quietly, get relaxed, then turn your hearing aid on as loud as you can stand it without being too uncomfortable. What do you hear? The sound of the furnace? Traffic going by? The hum of the refrigerator? Children playing outside? A dog barking? Listen to these sounds and try to identify each one. After a while, get up and walk around a bit. Does the chair squeak as you get up? How do your footsteps sound? Turn on the water faucet and listen to the swish of the water and the gurgling sound it makes as it goes down the drain. Listen to the sounds as you open and close a door, flush the stool, pull the drapes, read the newspaper. All of this may seem unimportant, but you haven't heard these sounds for some time, and if you don't get reused to them gradually, they'll bother you when you start listening to speech. Keep your volume control turned up as much as you can for as long as you can.

What if I start feeling nervous and fidgety? Then it's time to turn the aid down to a more comfortable level and wear it at this level for as long as you can. You may read or do anything else that isn't too noisy during this time. When the instrument starts to annoy you at this reduced level of loudness, turn it off, but keep it in your ear. When you're relaxed again, turn it back on for a short time longer. Finally, when the earpiece begins to bother, take the whole thing off, and put it away until you feel rested and ready to try it again. You'll find that you can wear it a little longer each time. Generally, the more you use the aid at first, the sooner you'll like it, but don't try to rush things to the point that you become overly irritated.

When can I start using my aid for talking to people? Not until you can wear it turned on fairly loud for an hour or two without conversation. By the time you can do this, you'll be used to background noises, so they won't distract you from listening attentively to speech. Don't try to converse with more than one person at a time at first. Begin with that person about six feet away from you, and adjust the volume control so you can *just* hear him comfortably. Ask him to speak in a normal voice and rather slowly. If you can understand him reasonably well at this distance, have him move a little farther away. You may need to turn the volume up a little as distance increases, but don't get in the habit of fiddling with the controls continually. After all, it's not possible to turn normal hearing up or down, so why make a fetish of doing it with your hearing aid?

I should be ashamed to tell you this, but the following ancecdote fits in so well with the above point that I can't resist. My college political science teacher wore a hearing aid, and one day in the spring when we were due for a quiz, the class decided to distract him a bit. When he walked in the door, we were all moving our lips and pretending to be talking, though we weren't making a sound. He looked startled and then started fumbling with his hearing aid controls. When we were sure he had it turned on full volume, we suddenly started talking in extra loud voices, which, of course, sent him scrimmaging for the controls again. (*Terrible* kids!) When he realized what was going on, he threw back his head and burst out in a loud guffaw. We knew he was a good sport, or we probably wouldn't have done it. Maybe you'll forgive me for taking part in such a fiendish plot if I plead that I was "too young to know better." (P.S. We *still* had the quiz!)

The point I'm trying to make is that it's best to find a comfortable level of loudness and keep the volume set there except when there is a significant change in listening conditions.

When I've learned to manage a one-to-one conversation passably, what's the next step? It's a tough one: learning to participate in group conversations. It's a little like trying to watch all three acts at the circus. Even with normal hearing, we don't hear everyone at once in a group conversation. We rapidly shift our attention from one person to another as each one speaks. This is especially difficult for the hard-of-hearing person, particularly if he wears a hearing aid in only one ear, because it's *binaural* (two-ear) hearing that tells us what direction sounds are coming from. If a person with normal hearing closes his eyes and listens to a group of people talking, he can point to each speaker as the conversation moves back and forth among the members of the group. A person with lopsided hearing, however, has to keep scanning the group visually till he discovers who is speaking. By the time he places the speaker, someone else probably has the floor, and he begins to wonder if it's worth the effort. If this happens to you, the best thing to do is to single out one person in the group who seems to be leading the conversation (*someone* always does) and stay focused on his speech. You will still miss some things, but this is better than trying to catch every pass and fumbling them all. I might as well say it: You may never reach the point of being really comfortable in group conversations, but if you develop the habit of concentrating on one speaker, you'll find that you'll at least get along better in those situations with your hearing aid than you would without it.

What about wearing my hearing aid away from home? Do not take the hearing aid out of the house until you've reached a satisfactory level of adjustment in the situations described above. Then, when you leave the house, you may have to turn the volume down a little, especially if you are going to be exposed to traffic noises. When you get to your destination, readjust the controls to a comfortable position.

Begin by wearing your aid when visiting in the homes of friends and relatives. When you're comfortable with that, you can wear it out in public, even though background noise will annoy you, especially at

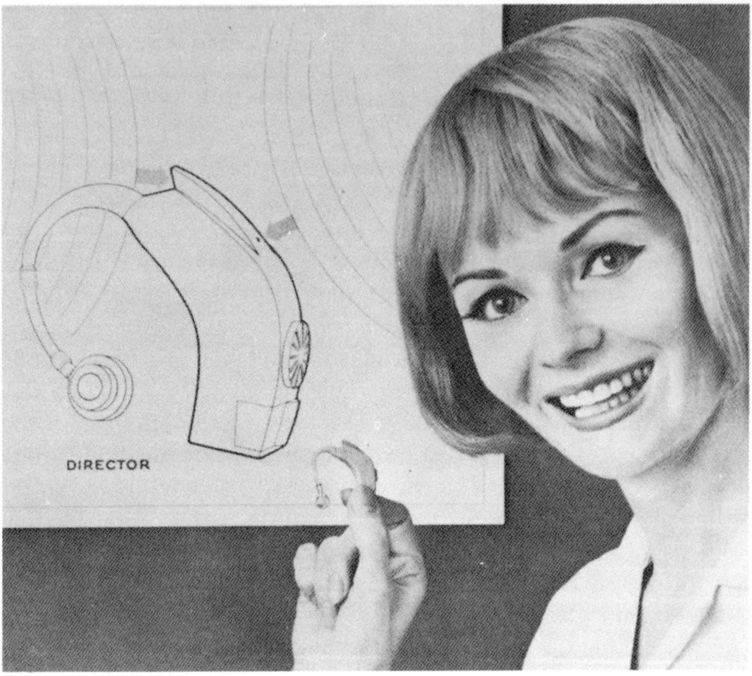

Figure 8.1. A typical directional-type hearing aid that amplifies sound coming from in front of the wearer while minimizing background noise coming from behind the wearer. (Courtesy of Zenith Hearing Instrument Corporation, a subsidiary of Zenith Radio Corporation.)

first. A directional hearing aid, such as the one shown in Figure 8.1, helps to cut down on extraneous sounds. When you do go to public places, you may want to try sitting in different parts of the auditorium, theater, church, or restaurant to discover the location in which you hear best. Before you go, give yourself a little pep talk. Be prepared for the fact that some of the sounds you hear will be strange, useless, and bothersome. If you're a fisherman, you've learned to put up with a few mosquito bites, an occasional dusty wind, even a sudden shower. When you come home with a good catch, you forget all about these nuisances. So go ahead and go to that movie, or to church, or to the concert. Go ahead and try out that new pizza parlor or steak house. The "catch" you come home with may be a better frame of mind, a more positive outlook on life.

Is it all right to turn the aid down or take it off when there's nothing

I especially want to hear? Don't get in the habit of doing this. If you turn the aid on only when you want to hear something special, there will be a certain amount of "auditory shock" each time you "tune in," and this will make it hard for you to concentrate on what you *want* to hear. Get used to wearing it as much as possible, and you and your "helper" will soon become good friends.

How long will my hearing aid last? The average life of a hearing aid is about three to five years, depending on the original quality of the instrument and the care you take of it. This may seem rather shocking to you, since we're talking about a fairly expensive piece of equipment. There's more than one reason, though, for replacing your hearing aid periodically. First, rapid advances in technology are constantly improving the quality, adaptability, and convenience of hearing aid design. In a few years, you may be able to get an aid that will make your hearing ability much closer to normal than your present one does. Then, too, your hearing itself may change, so that your present aid will be inadequate. At any rate, you should have a performance check of your aid at least once a year.

How much general overhead will there be in the operation of my hearing aid? Herman G. Wallenfels, author of *Hearing Aids for Nerve Deafness,* provides a good run-down on this:

> Battery cost is figured on hours-of-use basis. Calculating an average day to be fifteen hours, that is from seven in the morning until ten at night, the average consumer will need one package of batteries in a month. This would mean less than three dollars worth. You should also figure on an earmold tubing replacement once or twice a year at about one dollar and twenty-five cents each and a factory overhaul once a year after the second year. A hearing aid has many wearing parts. Same as an automobile, it will not perform as well as it should if it is permitted to deteriorate.[2]

How can I prolong the life of my hearing aid? It's surprising how much abuse these complicated and delicate electrical instruments can take, but don't invite trouble, as my little nephew did. He set out to prove that unbreakable phonograph records *aren't,* and he succeeded. He also succeeded in getting a very warm bottom! Of course, you're not going to try to find your aid's breaking point, but there are some things you can do to keep it in good working condition.

The receiver cord on a body-worn aid is the most vulnerable part. Always position the aid so there is some slack in this cord, and it will last longer. It's a good idea to keep a spare cord because it will probably have to be replaced, and those pesky things have a talent for giving out at the worst possible times.

Another common problem is created when perspiration seeps into the instrument, making it temporarily inoperative. To avoid this, insert a sheet of waterproofing material between the hearing aid case and your body.

If you're going to be engaging in vigorous activity while using a body-worn hearing aid, it's a good idea to use a belt or strap to hold the case in place so it won't get jarred too violently.

No matter what type of aid you have, the earpiece needs to be cleaned regularly with soap and warm water to keep wax from plugging it up. You can use a pipe cleaner for getting the sound channel clean. Be sure to dry the earpiece carefully and then blow through it to make certain you get every drop of water out. Keeping your earpiece clean will also help to prevent infection from developing in the ear canal.

What if the earpiece makes my ear sore? A little petroleum jelly smoothed over it may help. If not, take it back to the dealer, and he can buff it down to smooth out any rough places. If the ear insert seems to be moist when you take it out, an irritation may be present, and it's wise to have your otologist examine your ear. Don't ever use any medication in your ear without consulting him. Even cotton on a stick can be too rough, so obviously you must *never* insert such things as bobby pins or match sticks into your ear canal. There's a little sequence on the children's TV show "Sesame Street" that's appropriate here. A small cartoon character is scratching his ear with a stick of some kind, and another character says, "You should never put anything in your ear. It might damage your hearing," and the first little fellow yells, "WHAAT???!!"

Why does my ear itch? Some people are sensitive to the earmold plastics. It even happens, sometimes, that an intolerance for the plastic develops after a person has been wearing an earmold for years. You may want to have a new earmold made of nonallergic materials.

I can see that the suggestions in this chapter should help people who are trying to adjust to hearing aids, but aren't there some people who really don't want to hear better? Hearing impairment often brings with it a feeling of depression and hopelessness. When you're brooding, it's easy to decide that what you *would* hear if you *could* hear has no appeal for you, no meaning, no value. You may even welcome deafness as an excuse for not responding to the people around you. If you feel this way, don't add guilt to your already heavy load of mental anguish. Don't chide yourself for your attitude. Instead, recognize it for what it is: a very common, but usually temporary, reaction to your physical impairment. Then you'll realize that anything you can do to minimize that physical impairment will help pull you out of your fall into hopelessness. Getting a hearing aid may be just the rope you need to climb to get yourself out of that pit of despair.[3]

9 How can I learn to lipread?

"No, I can't lipread at all, and I really don't think I could learn, at my age."

Mrs. G. was sixty-two years old and had a severe sensori-neural hearing loss. She wore a hearing aid but still had quite a bit of difficulty understanding speech in many situations. As she sat across the desk from me, I placed my hand in front of my mouth and said in a soft voice, "I think you might be surprised at how much lipreading you already do."

She leaned forward and squinted. "What did you say?"

I then moved my hand so that she could see my lips and repeated, in the same quiet voice, "I think you might be surprised at how much lipreading you already do."

This time she understood easily and replied, "Oh. Really?"

Again, I placed my hand in front of my lips and asked, "Are you sure you can't lipread at all?"

The strained look came back to her face. "What did you say?"

Again I repeated my question, this time without obstructing her view of my lips. She laughed as she began to understand the point I was trying to prove. "Well, I guess I *can* understand better when I can see your lips. But that isn't really lipreading, is it? I'm still using my hearing, too."

Many people believe, as Mrs. G. did, that lipreading is a special skill that's completely separated from hearing. I saw a movie once in which a detective hired a "lipreading expert" to look through binoculars into an office window across the street and tell him what the people were saying. He did it, too. Word for word. It could only happen in the movies, believe me!

Actually, only about a third of all speech sounds are *clearly* visible on the lips. So word-for-word "translation," especially without *any* sound, would be impossible, even for the best lipreader. Lipreading is a tool that can help you fill in the gaps your impaired hearing creates. It is a *supplement* to whatever hearing you have left. The greater the amount of your loss, the more you need to depend on your vision to hold up your communication bridges. As people begin to lose their hearing, they unconsciously begin to use their eyes to make up for what their ears miss.

Like Mrs. G., you probably already have some skill in lipreading. You can demonstrate this for yourself by having a friend or relative say something to you in a soft voice, with his hand in front of his mouth and, if you can't hear it, having him repeat it in the same quiet voice while you watch his lips.

If, as you say, I already lipread, why do I need training in it? Your ability to lipread can be very much increased by conscious awareness and practice on your part. Also, if your hearing loss should become worse, you'll be able to cope much better if you already understand and use the principles that make for effective lipreading.

What's the difference between lipreading and speechreading? Both terms refer to the same thing. Actually, speechreading is a more accurate word because the visual clues you'll be using are not limited to the lips. Gestures, body position, facial expression, situational clues, and many other visual factors affect your ability to use your eyes to help your ailing ears. I've decided to use the term lipreading in this book, though, because it's more commonly known.

Which should come first, auditory training or lipreading? Actually, they should not be separated. Studies have shown that the best approach to hearing rehabilitation is a *multisensory* approach. In other words, you should try to make the best possible use of all your senses, letting each one reinforce the others as much as possible. Mark Ross notes that "the literature frequently treats lipreading and auditory training as if they were separate entities. In practice, however, the two procedures interweave; sometimes they are practiced separately, sometimes simultaneously. . . ."[1] When you're practicing at home, you'll sometimes want to combine hearing practice (see Chapter 10) with lipreading practice. At other times, you'll do them separately, but always remember that your goal is to improve your ability to communicate and that, to do that, you'll need to use *all* of your senses to their fullest.

I've heard there are different methods for learning to lipread.

Which one is best? Many different systems have been developed, but most of them fall into one of three categories: (1) the analytic method, (2) the synthetic method, and (3) a combination of the two. In the analytic method, you begin by studying single sounds, such as the *p* sound, then work up to syllables, then words, then sentences, and finally paragraphs or conversation. A major drawback in this method is that, when sounds are run together in speech, they look different from the way they look by themselves. Also, some sounds, such as the *k* and *g* sounds, have no *visible* characteristics, so the only way the lipreader can tell whether the word being used is *coat* or *goat* is by listening to the rest of the sentence.

What's the synthetic method? Advocates of this system believe that, since understanding *thoughts* is what counts, the lipreader should practice extracting meaning from whole sentences and conversational speech without being concerned about individual sounds. Let's call this procedure *thought-unit practice.*

How does the combination method work? Obviously, this method uses both single-sound practice and thought-unit practice for developing lipreading skills. Most lipreading teachers today prefer this approach. Later in this chapter I'll give you suggestions for your home practice based on this combination.

Is there anything I need to do before I begin lipreading practice? Of course, you'll need to have a thorough physical and audiological evaluation of your hearing and to follow through on any recommendations your doctor or audiologist makes. If these professional people recommend a hearing aid, you'll want to wait until you've adjusted reasonably well to your new aid before you begin to study lipreading.

Also, how long has it been since you've had your eyes examined? It's very important for you to see as well as possible in order to get the most out of lipreading. So check up on your vision and have it corrected to whatever extent is possible.

Can I teach myself to lipread? Well, if a speech and hearing clinician is available, he can help you a great deal, but even then, you'll need to practice on your own, too. Olive Wyatt, in her book *Teach Yourself Lip-reading,* says:

> . . . I would suggest that most of the work must be done by yourself in practice, anywhere and everywhere. While I would in no way decry formal study under a trained teacher, I must emphasize that it is this constant practice that does most of the teaching; it encourages learners to be their own

> teachers in always trying to find out the how, why and wherefore of the thing. All that we need for teaching ourselves lip-reading is a little courage and common sense and a good deal of spirit and perseverance, and the facility will "come".[2]

If a speech and hearing clinician or a lipreading class is available in your area, by all means take advantage of that opportunity. If not, it will be very helpful to you if you can recruit a member of your family or a friend to be your helper in some phases of your home training. Maybe you have a hard-of-hearing friend. If so, the two of you can work together on lipreading and help each other. Here are some suggestions for the person who will be helping you.

Notes to your helper. Do not try to form words without using your voice when you are providing lipreading practice for your hard-of-hearing friend. It is almost impossible for most people to keep their speech movements natural when they try to mouth words without voice. Instead, have the hearing-impaired person remove his hearing aid, and then you speak in a soft voice.

Do not exaggerate your speech movements. This only makes it more difficult for your friend to lipread.

Do speak slowly, especially in the beginning. Later, after your friend becomes more proficient at lipreading, you can increase your speaking to a normal conversational speed.

Experts have found that about six to ten feet between speaker and lipreader works best. Try out different distances until you find the one that's most comfortable for him and gives the best results.

Don't chew gum or smoke while you're helping your friend practice lipreading. It will make lipreading twice as hard for him. If you're a woman, wear a bright shade of lipstick for these sessions. If you're a man with a mustache, do you think you could bear to part with it for the sake of the person you're helping? If not, do keep it trimmed as closely as possible.

And—just from me to you—thanks so much for helping my hard-of-hearing friend!

Do I need any special equipment? Not anything you don't already have. You *will* need a well-lighted room. The source of light should always come from *behind* you, so that it will illuminate the face of the person whose lips you're reading or make your own face clearer if you're practicing with a mirror by yourself. Also, with the light behind you, you won't need to worry about glare, which would make it harder for you to see. Then you'll need a good mirror—either the vanity, hand-held type or one on an easel that will stand by itself on the table. Some exercises require the use of a notebook or tablet. Any kind will do. If you have a TV set, you will be able to use it for some assignments, and a record player or tape recorder would be handy for providing background distraction in later lessons, but it's not necessary. I'll be mentioning some books that will be helpful to you in various phases of your lipreading practice. They may be available from your public library or from a nearby college library or from a speech and hearing clinic in your area. Or you may order them from the publisher if you feel you can afford to buy them. There are also some mail-order lending libraries for the hearing handicapped. Write to Duane King, Deaf Missions, Route 2, Council Bluffs, IA 51501. The people there are very nice, and they'll send you any book or books on their list for two weeks, without charge. They do hope that those who can afford to will send a free-will offering so that those who can't afford to pay can use the materials without charge. They are providing a fine, unselfish service for hearing-impaired people.

Should I use my hearing aid during lipreading practice? There will be times when you'll use it at normal setting, other times when I'll ask you to turn the volume down, and still other practice situations in which you should turn it off or remove it completely. I'll tell you about these as we proceed through the lessons.

Should I set aside a certain period of time every day for lipreading practice? It would be helpful to do this. Otherwise, if you're like I am, you'll always be *intending* to get to it! Choose a time of day when you're likely to be relaxed and rested and not rushed. Plan to work on lipreading when there won't be too many distractions. *But*—treat this as a hobby. Don't grit your teeth and tense up and *force* yourself to keep after it until you're all worn out. Let the way you *feel* determine how much time you spend at each session. If you feel yourself getting tired and frustrated, STOP and do something else.

Where do I begin? The suggestions I'm going to give you for improving your lipreading ability fall into five general categories. We'll call them Groups A, B, C, D, and E. Try to choose one project from each group every week. For example, you could choose to work on something from Group A on Monday, Group B on Tuesday, etc. After some weeks of practicing these, you will be able to think up similar exercises of your own.

What is the purpose of group A? As I said earlier, lipreading involves much more than just watching people's lips. Some people learn to lipread much more easily than others do. Experts who've studied these differences have found that people who are naturally observant progress more rapidly. This is an ability that can be developed, so let's begin with some exercises to improve your visual awareness.

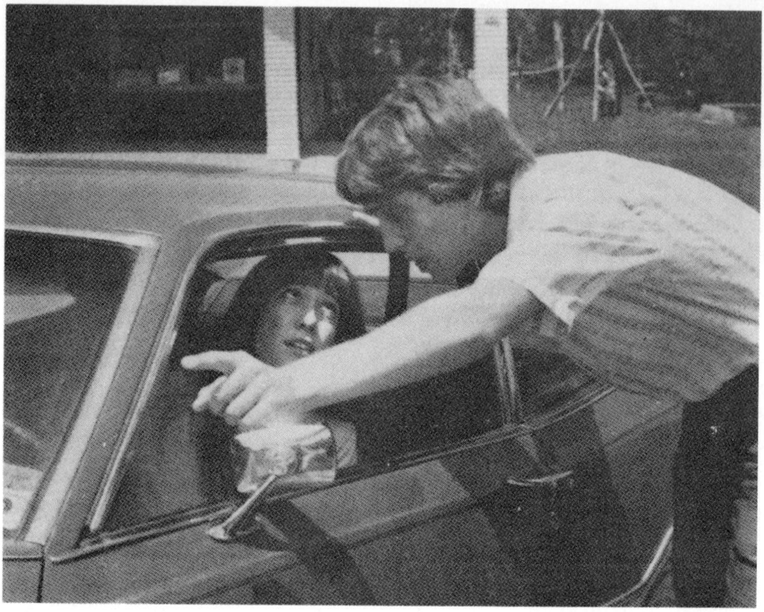

Figure 9.1. Practice sizing up situations by watching people's actions. Some gestures, such as pointing, beckoning, and waving, have universal meanings. Visual clues let you know immediately what is going on in the above picture.

Group A. Visual awareness 1. Take a little tablet or notebook with at least fifteen pages in it and write down, on five separate pages, the names of five people you see frequently. Leave three pages between names. On the first page write (from memory) a brief description of the facial features of each one. (E.g., Aunt Emmy has a broad nose and crooked teeth. Friend Bill has squinty eyes and frown lines and always looks as if he needs a shave.) Then turn the page and list some of the personal mannerisms of each. (Joe chews gum constantly. Sally's face gets red when she's angry. Pat usually sits with her arms folded across her chest.) Go to the next page and list the favorite topics of conversation of each person on your list. Be sure to do all this from memory.

Now. Each time you see one of these people, try to find something to add to your list. You'll be surprised how many things you'll discover that you'd never noticed before. This will help you get in the habit of being visually observant.

2. Page through the illustrations in a magazine and see if you can tell, without reading the captions, what the articles or stories are about. Do the same thing with pictures in the newspaper.

3. If you have a TV set, tune in to a soap opera and turn the sound down as far as it will go. Watch the actors' facial expressions, gestures, and movements about the room and see if you can determine what emotions they're portraying. (Joy? Surprise? Worry? Anger?) Then turn the sound up (and your hearing aid, too, if necessary) to see if you're right.

4. On another day, repeat the soap opera routine, but this time, see how much you can tell about the characters themselves by observing their clothing and hair styles, room decor, objects in the room, etc. How old are they? Are they rich, poor, or in between? Can you tell by watching their actions what their relationships to one another are? Husband and wife, father and son, lovers, friends? You'll find that this kind of practice will carry over into your daily life by helping you to quickly size up the situation whenever you walk into a room. The more information you can get by making quick observations, the better prepared you'll be for following any conversation.

5. Keep a list of gestures and mannerisms you notice your family and friends using. Write after each one what you think the gesture means. (E.g., Dad puts his hands on his hips when he's angry. Sister picks at her hangnails when she's nervous.) What does a shrug indicate? A sudden toss of the head? A stomp of the foot? If you get in the habit of "reading" gestures and mannerisms, you can pick up some valuable clues about what's being said.

6. Get a good book on nonverbal communication, or as it's sometimes called, body language, and study it carefully. Some good examples are: *Beyond Words,* by Randall P. Harrison (Englewood Cliffs, N.J.: Prentice-Hall, 1974); and *Silent Messages,* by Albert Mehrabian (Belmont, Calif.: Wadsworth Publishing Co., 1971). Look under *nonverbal*

communication in the card catalog of your library for other books on this subject.

What is included in group B? Another ability that has been repeatedly found in good lipreaders is a strong *visual memory span.* This means that they can hold a picture in their minds for a while even when they can no longer see the actual object.

Why is this important in lipreading? Remember that you're not going to be able to lipread *every* word in most spoken sentences. And sometimes, you're not going to be sure about a particular word until the speaker comes to the end of a sentence. So you'll often need to be able to remember the speech movements you see *early* in a sentence until the speaker has completed his thought. Then you can put the pieces together in your mind and come up with a meaningful interpretation. Like the visual awareness of Group A, your visual memory span can be stretched.

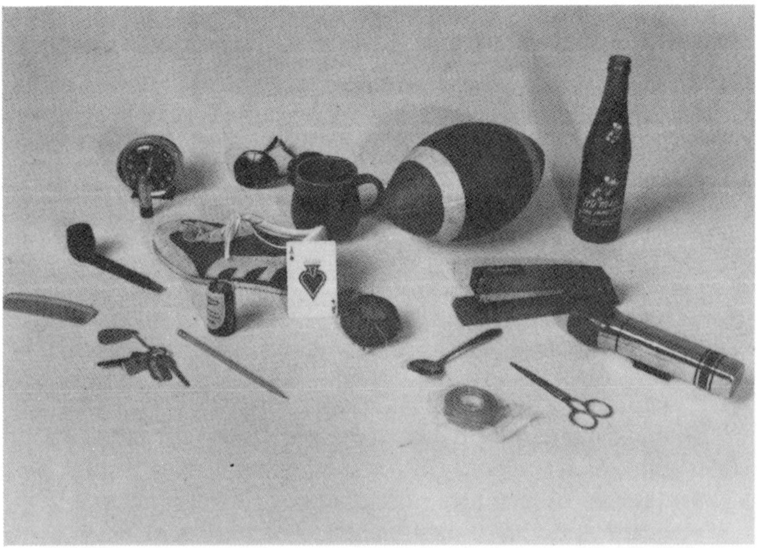

Figure 9.2. Memorize these items to help increase your visual memory span. Or use a picture in a magazine.

Group B. Visual memory span. 1. Look at the picture in Figure 9.2 for one minute. Have someone time you, or set your stove timer. Then close the book, and write down as many items as you can remember. You can also do this with pictures in magazines, trying to recall as many details as possible. You'll find your ability to do this increasing with practice. Your visual memory span will be growing!

2. Watch a television newscast in the morning or at noon, with the TV sound and your hearing aid turned up as high as necessary for you to hear to the best of your ability. Then watch another newscast later in the same day (6:00 or 10:00 P.M. or whenever it's convenient.) But this time, do it without your hearing aid and with the TV audio turned down. Since many of the news items you heard earlier in the day will be repeated, you'll be using your memory to help you lipread. How many of the news items could you identify? Try to increase that number the next time you try this exercise.

3. Derek Sanders suggests having someone place a number of objects on a table or tray, covered with a towel.[3] Lift the towel and look at the objects for twenty seconds; then recover them and see how many you can recall. Start with ten items and increase the number each time you repeat this exercise in future sessions.

4. As a variation of the above, ask your friend to *remove* one item after you've studied them and then see if you can determine which object is missing.

5. Write the numbers from one to ten, in several different sequences, on separate pages of your notebook. (E.g., 6, 2, 5, 10, 1, 4, 8, 7, 9, 3.) Choose a page and read the sequence through *once*. Then close your eyes and try to repeat it correctly.

6. The following exercise is for use after you have learned to recognize the lip movements of the numbers from one to ten. Remove your hearing aid and ask your helper to say these ten numbers out of sequence in a soft voice. He should write them down so you can check to see if you've repeated them correctly.

7. Do Exercise 6 using days of the week, months of the year, etc.

What skills are developed by the exercises in group C? Since you won't be able to lipread every word, you'll need to develop your ability to fill in the gaps. The experts call this ability *closure*. Sanders defines it as "the tendency we have to perceive an incomplete figure as being complete. It accounts, in part, for the ability of a person to recognize a spoken word or sentence on the basis of limited visual cues, or for a person with a marked hearing loss correctly to perceive certain sounds that are inaudible to him."[4] For instance, you might lipread the following words from your wife, who is standing in the kitchen doorway: "John, ——— ready ——— eat. Please ——— ——— children ——— wash ——— ———." You'll probably be able to fill in the words you missed. ("John, we're ready to eat. Please tell the children to wash their hands.") Again, you can greatly increase your ability to fill in gaps by practicing, so the exercises in Group C are directed toward that end.

Group C. Closure. 1. Ask your helper to write down several sentences, leaving out a word from each one and putting a blank (———) in its place. Try to fill in the blanks. If you don't come up with the exact word he had in mind, it doesn't matter, as long as your word makes sense in the sentence.

2. Have your helper do the same thing with a whole paragraph, omitting at least one word in each sentence. This time, the words you put in must make sense in the context of the whole paragraph.

3. Read a short story in a magazine, but stop several paragraphs before the end. Try to figure out how the story ends. Then finish reading it.

4. Ask your helper to cut out five cartoons from newspapers or magazines and then cut off and save the captions. First, try to decide what each caption might be, just by looking at the cartoons alone. Then take the captions and lay them out on the table under the cartoons and try to match them up. You'll find that your growing ability to *predict* what's coming will help you to think ahead in real life lipreading situations. If you can form some idea of what a person *might* say in a given situation, you'll be more likely to understand him when he does talk.

5. If you understand manual communication (or sign language), watch one of the TV programs that provide signing along with the regular program. ("The Christophers" on Sunday morning on CBS is a program of this type.) Remove your hearing aid and turn the TV audio off. Now watch the lips of the person *speaking* and try to follow what he is saying. Refer to the person who is "signing" down in the corner of the picture only when you become lost. At first, you'll probably need to rely on the signer quite often, but try to increase the amount of understanding you can gain by watching the speaker's lips.

6. Your ability to make closure involves skill in picking out what's important and ignoring the rest. So practice reading a paragraph in a book, magazine, or newspaper and then try to summarize the central idea in a single sentence.

7. Games such as Anagrams and Scrabble, jigsaw puzzles, and scrambled word games (e.g., the "Jumble" that's printed in many newspapers) also help to increase one's ability to make closure.

What is group D? The exercises in this category will make you conscious of the visual movements associated with specific sounds and combinations of sounds.

Group D. Individual sounds and words. 1. For this exercise, you'll need your mirror and your notebook. Use your hearing aid, turned up to your best level for hearing. When we start to study the lip movements the various sounds make, we discover that many of them, such as *p, b,* and *m,* look alike. List the following groupings in your notebook, leaving several spaces between groups:

m, b, p
f, v
th, l
sh, ch, j
s, z
t, d, n
w, wh

Now start with the first group *(p, b, m).* Follow steps a., b., c., and d. with this group now. On another day, follow the same four steps with the second group of sounds *(f, v),* and so on, taking only one sound group at a session.

a. Look in your mirror and say the sound the letter makes. It's very important, at this point, that you understand the difference between *naming the letter* and making the *sound* of it. In other words, don't say "em, bee, pee." Just form the *sound* that the letter would make if it appeared in a word. If this difference still isn't clear to you, say a word beginning with the letter, such as 'm*other*.' Then just leave off the *'other'* and say the sound, *'m,'* by itself.

As you watch yourself making the sounds in your mirror, ask yourself what movements of your lips, teeth, and tongue you can *see.* Write down your description of these visible movements.

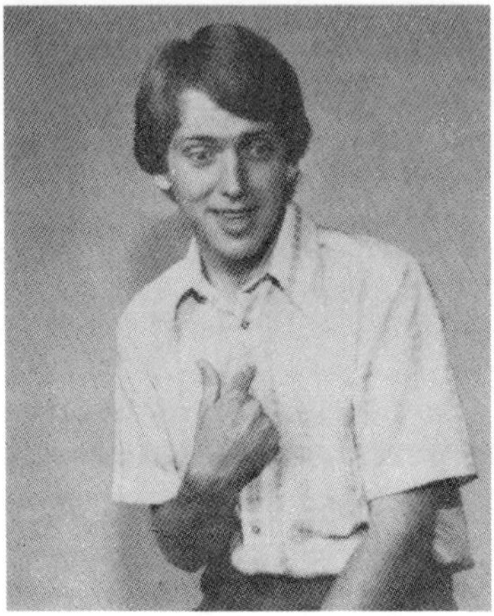

a

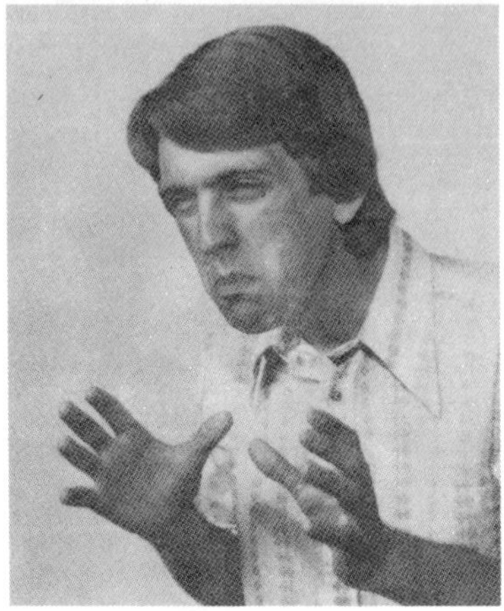

b

Figure 9.3. Try to become more aware of the meanings you can pick up from facial expressions and gestures. See if you can match the following captions to the correct pictures above. 1. "And there it was, *crawling* across my plate!" 2. "Well, I surely have enjoyed hearing about your operation, *but* . . . 3. "*I* know who we can get to volunteer for the cleanup committee—you!" 4. "You think *I* ate the last piece?" 5. "Wait'll I get my hands on that guy. I'll . . . I'll. . . ." 6. "Now, open your mouth and close your eyes, and I'll give you a big surprise."

ANSWERS: 1-d; 2-f; 3-e; 4-a; 5-b; 6-c.

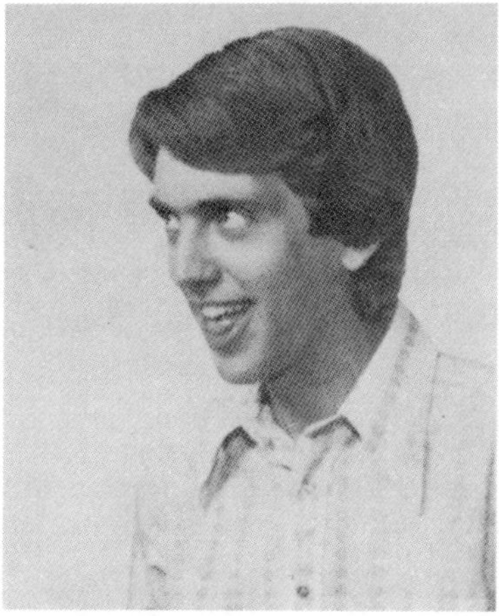

c

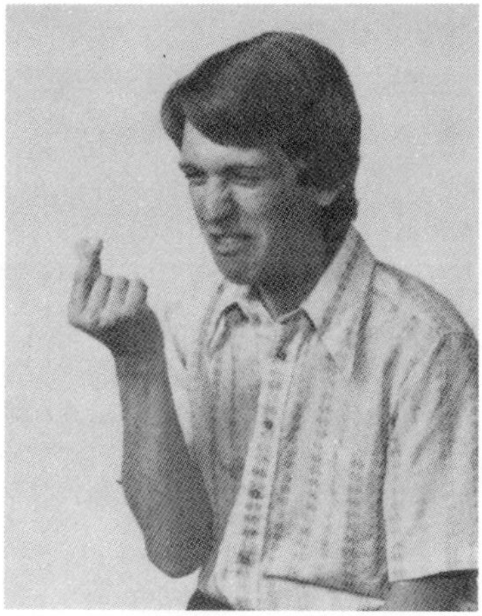

d

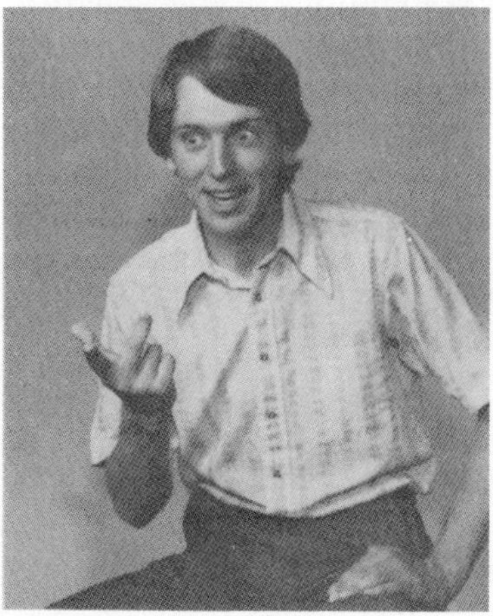

e

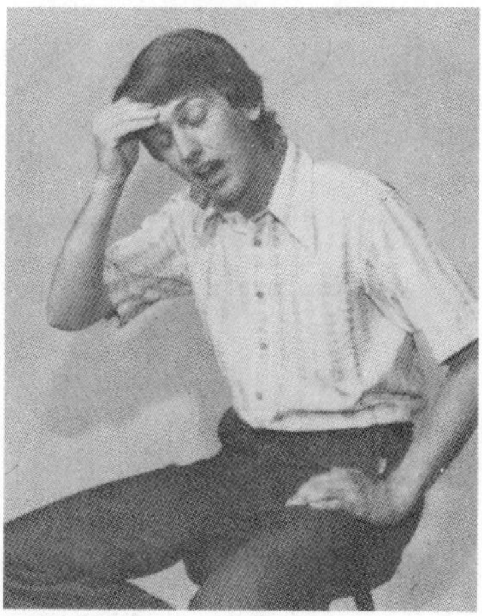

f

b. Now compare your descriptions with those listed in Table 9.1.

Table 9.1. Visible Movements of Consonant Sounds

p,b,m	Lips are pressed together and then released.
f,v	Lower lip touches upper front teeth, then returns to open position.
th,l	Tongue can be seen protruding slightly between upper and lower teeth.
sh, ch,j	Lips are slightly rounded and projected outward.
s,z	Corners of mouth are pulled back slightly, as in a faint smile. Teeth, barely apart, can be seen through lip opening.
t,d,n	Lips are open in a relaxed position. It is sometimes possible to see the tip of the tongue, which is raised and touching the roof of the mouth behind the upper teeth.
w,wh	Lips are rounded, with only a small center opening.

c. Next, repeat the sound group again, paying particular attention to how the sounds *feel* as you say them. You are now combining the sense of hearing (your aid is still turned up, isn't it?) and vision (be sure to use your mirror) and touch (the way the sound *feels* on your tongue, lips, and teeth.) Each of these senses will reinforce the others to stamp the visual impression firmly in your mind.

d. Now, using the same sound group, practice saying words that begin with each sound, to see how the movement looks, sounds, and feels in words. (E.g., *p*an, *b*oy, *m*ope). Then do the same with words that have the sounds in the middle position (u*p*on, a*b*le, co*m*mon). Finally, try words that end with the sounds (u*p*, glo*b*e, hu*m*). Repeat steps a, b, c, and d with the next sound group *(f, v)* the next time you do this exercise (on another day).

Once you learn to recognize the movements associated with each sound *group,* the meaning of the sentence will help you determine which letter of a particular group makes sense. For instance, in the sentence 'She put the pan on the stove burner,' it's not likely that you'll confuse *pan* with *man*.

2. Choose an article or story that interests you and read it through. Then ask your helper to pick out one paragraph from the selection. Remove your hearing aid and have him read the paragraph to you in a quiet voice. Now tell him, in your own words, what the paragraph was about. If you get lost during the reading, have him stop and repeat that part slowly. It may help you to silently 'mimic' his speech move-

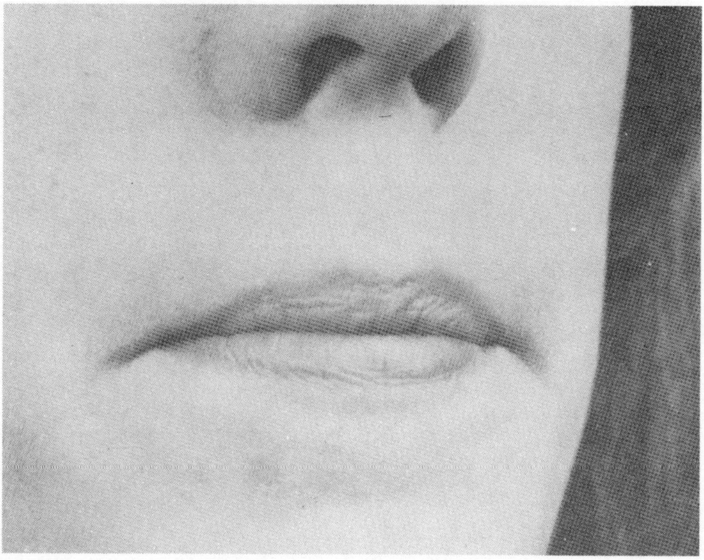

Figure 9.4. The *p, b,* and *m* sounds are the only ones in which there is complete lip closure.

Figure 9.5. When the lower lip touches the upper teeth, the sound being formed is either *f* or *v*.

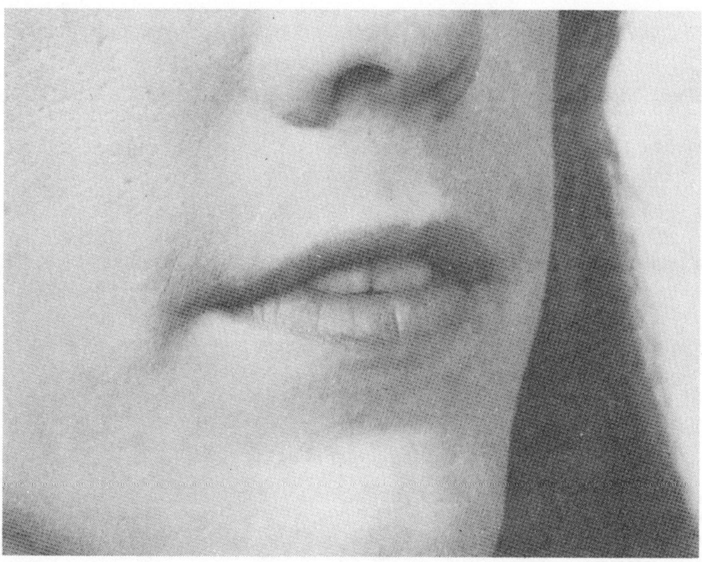

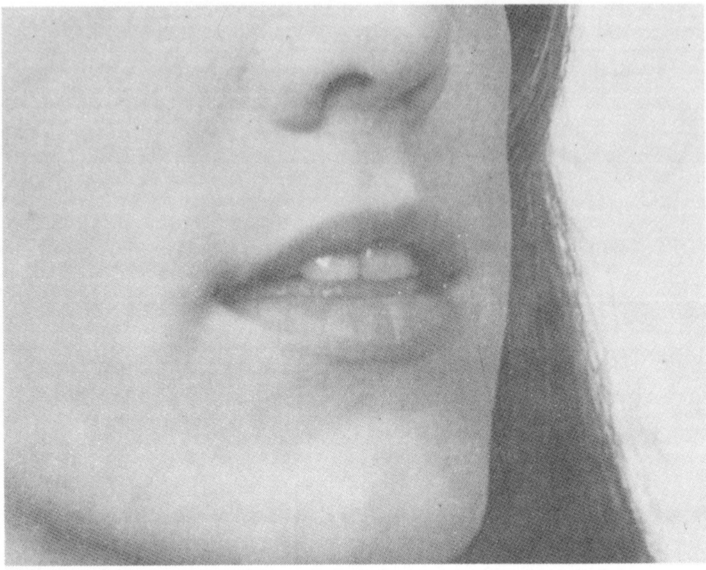

Figure 9.6. The tip of the tongue is usually visible between the teeth when the *th* and *l* sounds are formed.

Figure 9.7. Rounded and protruding lips will help you to identify the *sh, ch,* and *j* sounds.

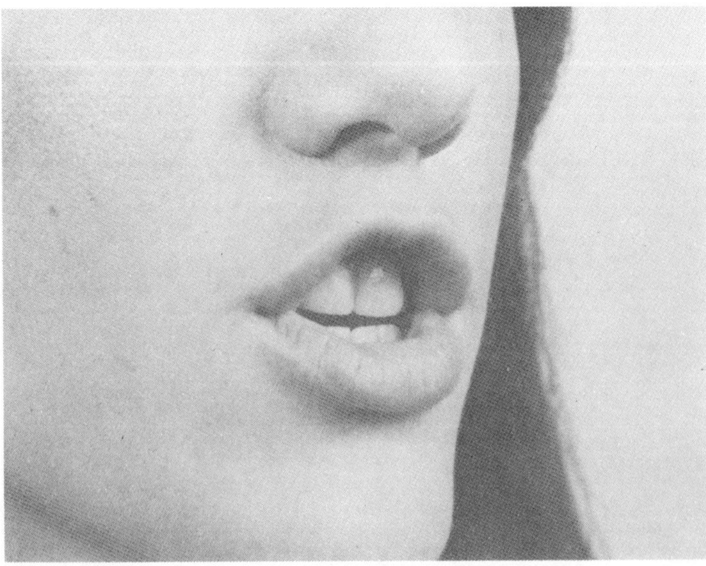

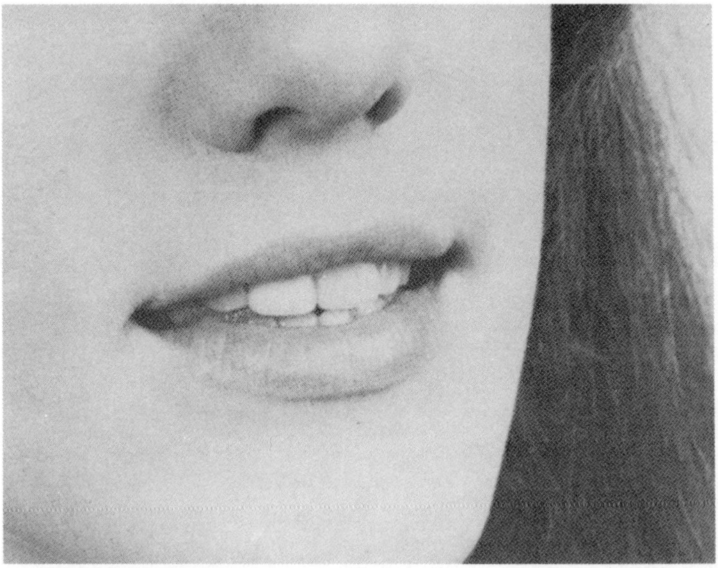

Figure 9.8. The position for the *s* and *z* sounds resembles a slight smile, with both upper and lower teeth visible.

Figure 9.9. A raised tongue is slightly visible during the production of the *l, d,* and *n* sounds.

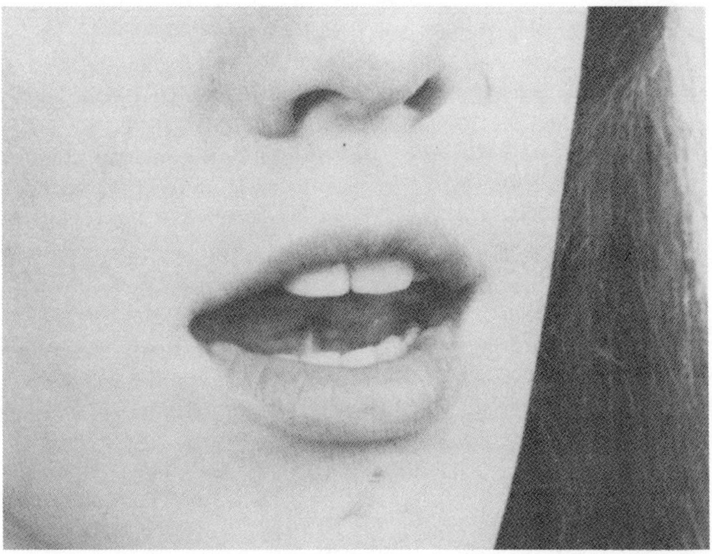

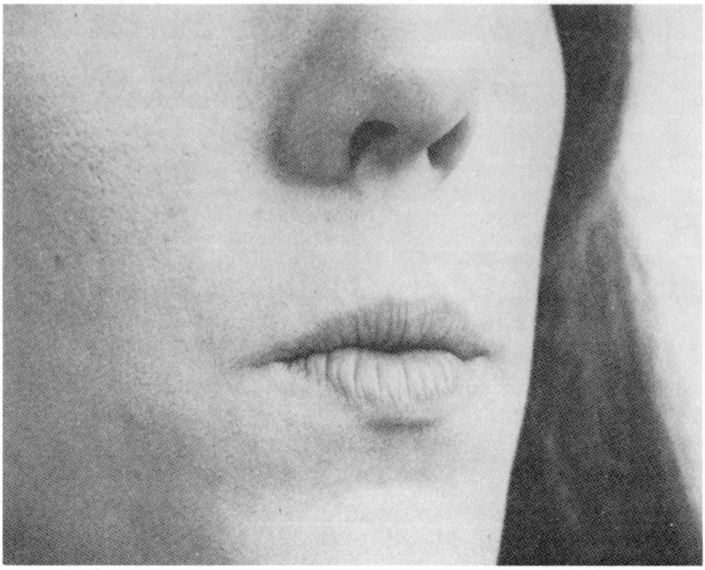

Figure 9.10. A marked rounding of the lips will help you to recognize the *w* and *wh* sounds.

ments yourself as he does so. (This is where the "feeling" practice of Exercise 1 comes to your aid.)

3. You'll soon learn which sounds you have the most difficulty with, so get an articulation practice book, such as *Fundamentals of Voice and Diction,* by Lyle V. Mayer. There are many others, and your audiologist or speech clinician may have one to loan you or will make suggestions for an appropriate practice book for you. Ask your helper to read practice material to you from the sections that cover your problem sounds. If your loss is severe, use your hearing aid for this practice so that you can combine both auditory and visual cues for understanding. After all, this is what you'll be doing in everyday life situations.

How can I use my lipreading skills to best advantage in everyday life? This is the purpose of the exercises in Group E.

Group E. Conversation skills. 1. First of all, be well informed. Read the newspaper every day. Watch and listen to TV newscasts. Ask family members to keep you informed about things that are happening in your community and neighborhood and about events in the lives of people you know.

2. Before you go to a party or meeting, see if you can find out who will be there. Learn as much about these people as you can (occupation, marital status, number of children, recent trips they may have taken, hobbies, etc.) This information will help you to predict possible topics of conversation and may make it possible for you to guide conversations to subjects that interest them. When you know the subject of a conversation, it's *much* easier to lipread!

3. There's an excellent manual that may be available at a nearby college library or from a speech and hearing clinic in your area. It's called *What People Say.* The book includes expressions that commonly are used in specific situations, such as what people say—

about the weather,
at the dinner table,
at election time,
at the movies,
about hearing aids,
upon leaving, etc.

If you can get a copy of this book, study it by yourself first, and then ask your helper to say the expressions under one category at a time as you lipread them.

4. If your hearing loss developed before you were an adult, get a good book of idioms from the library and study their uses. An idiom is a commonly used expression that has a special meaning that may be completely different from what the words themselves say. One idiom, for instance, is 'You sure let the cat out of the bag'; it doesn't have anything at all to do with cats. People use it to mean, 'You sure gave away the secret.' People with normal hearing pick up and use these expressions almost without realizing it, but idioms can be very puzzling and misleading to people who've always had trouble hearing.

5. Learn to control your lipreading environment. When you walk into a room where people are talking, try to seat yourself so the light (window, lamp, whatever) will come from behind you. Choose a chair that will allow you to be facing as many people as possible.

6. When you meet someone for the first time, don't hesi-

tate to tell him that you have a hearing loss. Tell him that you can understand him best if he'll speak in a normal voice and keep his face turned toward you. Since it's natural for people to look at one another's eyes when conversing, you may want to tell him that you lipread. This way, he'll understand why you're focusing on his lips instead of his eyes. Now, I know what you're thinking. You're too embarrassed to say these things to a stranger. Right? Would you rather have him think you're retarded? Believe me, it will relieve *both* of you if you'll let *this* "cat out of the bag"! You'll both be more at ease immediately. He'll respect you for being open and honest about your problem, and *now* the two of you can carry on a reasonable conversation, where as before it would have been difficult, if not impossible.

7. Conversations involving several people will always be one of your most difficult problems, but it will help you immensely if you can recruit your mate or a friend to give you cues. Ask him to get in the habit of letting you know whenever there's a change of subject. He can do this unobtrusively by turning to you and saying, "Ellen's daughter has been sick," or "Did you hear about the filling station robbery?" or "Pat has an antique car he likes to work on."

Another thing that will help you when you're in a group is to determine who seems to be leading the conversation. Usually, one person tends to take the lead, and if you find this is the case, keep your attention focused on his lips instead of trying to jump around from person to person as different people speak. Sure, you'll miss some comments this way, but it'll be less tiring for you, and you'll probably be able to keep track of the gist of the conversation *better.*

8. When you begin to feel confident about your lipreading ability, try practicing with some distraction. Turn on the TV or record player. Choose programs or records that involve speech (not just background music) because this provides the greatest distraction. This exercise will help you get used to focusing your attention on what you're trying to lipread and ignoring other sounds. It's an ability that will be valuable to you in many life situations, such as eating in a noisy restaurant, checking out at the grocery store, conversing on the bus or at parties, etc.

The Alexander Graham Bell Association for the Deaf has an extensive inventory of lipreading practice materials which can be of great help to you in your home study. I'd suggest you write to ask for their publication list. The address is: Alexander Graham Bell Association for the Deaf, Inc.; 3417 Volta Place, N.W.; Washington, D.C. 20007.

I think you can see, from reading the foregoing suggestions, that lipreading doesn't have to be tedious and boring. It can be challenging and fun. It should never be dull, day-after-day drill. The suggestions in this chapter will provide variety and a growing sense of accomplishment. Oh, I know you'll probably get discouraged sometimes and wonder if you're really getting anywhere. But, even when you can't *see* your progress, it's going on, nevertheless. If you'll just keep with it, you can't *help* but grow in your ability to lipread. Remember that the only people who never get discouraged are the ones who never try to accomplish anything.

10

What is auditory training and how can it help me?

Have you ever learned a skill that takes a great deal of practice, such as playing a musical instrument or typing? If so, you know that, when you get out of practice because you haven't used this skill regularly for a while, you become "rusty." In other words, the things that were once more or less *automatic* for you when you were practicing regularly now require conscious effort on your part. Using your hearing for understanding speech involves processes that have to be learned through listening practice. For the child with good hearing, this practice occurs unconsciously. But what happens if he develops a hearing loss later in life? Like the secretary who takes a few years off to raise a family and has to "brush up" on her typing to go back to work, the listening abilities of a hard-of-hearing adult deteriorate from lack of use. When he gets a hearing aid, he needs to "brush up" on his listening skills through practice. What was once automatic now requires a conscious effort and more practice. This is *one* of the purposes of auditory training.

Do you mean that, by practice, I can actually increase my hearing level? Not exactly. Auditory training won't improve your hearing threshold as measured by a pure-tone audiometer. But it *can* help you to better understand speech. Raymond Carhart defines it as "the process of teaching the child or adult who is hard of hearing to take full advantage of sound cues which are still available to him."[1] In other words, it's very likely that you are not now *using* the hearing you have to your best advantage. Auditory training, like lipreading, can help you learn to develop an awareness of cues that you may not be *noticing* now.

Auditory training takes various forms, depending on the severity of your loss and your age at the time of onset. For instance, the child who was *born* with a severe hearing loss needs to be taught how to attach meaning to the weak and distorted sound signals his ears pick up. He needs to learn that even the small amount of hearing he has can give him valuable cues about what's going on around him.

But what good will auditory training do for the person who develops a hearing loss later in life? When a person becomes hard of hearing, he automatically begins to pay more attention to the *visual* speech cues and less attention to the *sounds* of speech. If his hearing loss interferes greatly with his communication ability, he may unconsciously 'give up' and stop trying to listen. When this happens, a systematic program of auditory training can help to focus his attention again on the act of listening and on the auditory signals he's been largely ignoring.

Remember when I told you about losing part of my money on my way to the store to buy a kite? My first reaction was to give up because I knew that what I had left wasn't enough to buy the kite I wanted. But, with my parents' help, I learned that I could use the money I had left in a *different* way and still stay in the contest. In the same way, auditory training can help you to use the hearing you have left more effectively. If your hearing has been impaired for some time and you have recently acquired a hearing aid, auditory training can help you get back in the habit of listening. It can also help you learn to distinguish between the sounds that are still "too much alike," even with the help of your hearing aid. You will need to *relearn* several aspects of perception and discrimination. Later, auditory training can give you practice in separating speech sounds from distracting background noise—a valuable skill for the difficult day-to-day conversational situations you'll encounter.

There's another way that auditory training can help you with the sometimes difficult task of adjusting to a hearing aid. If you have a problem with recruitment—in other words, if loud sounds bother you a lot—the amount of amplification you can take is limited. You may have to keep your hearing aid turned down to a much lower setting than you require for good understanding of speech. Auditory training can help to gradually increase the amount of amplification you can comfortably use. Obviously, if you can learn to be comfortable with a higher level of amplification, your hearing aid can then serve you better by delivering more sound to your ears.

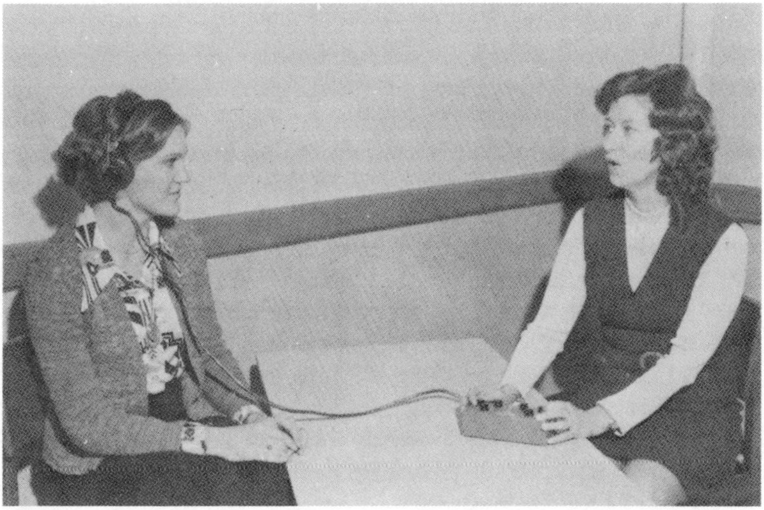

Figure 10.1. An auditory training unit, such as this one, delivers precise levels of amplification that can be adjusted separately for each ear. The unit provides an optimum listening situation for practice in sound discrimination and for increasing tolerance to amplification. In the picture above, the clinician is combining auditory training with lipreading practice in working with a hard-of-hearing girl.

Does every hard-of-hearing adult need auditory training? Newby gives us a good answer to this question:

> The adult with a hearing impairment which is easily compensated for by a hearing aid may require no auditory training, whereas an individual with a typical sensori-neural impairment, who has considerably better hearing in the low frequencies than in the high ones, will probably benefit from auditory training whether or not he wears a hearing aid. The test of whether or not auditory training is indicated is the individual's ability to *understand* speech with or without amplification.[2]

So, if you can understand speech well with your hearing aid, you probably don't need auditory training. The majority of hearing-impaired adults, though, do have sensori-neural losses, with greater losses in the higher frequencies and usually some recruitment problems. If your hearing loss is of this type, you're almost sure to benefit from auditory training.

Do I need professional help with it? If there is a speech and hearing clinic or clinician in your area, you would be wise to seek professional help. Professionals understand the principles involved and can tailor your training to fit your particular needs. They also have access to a desk-type auditory training unit. This type of equipment can provide better-quality sound transmission than your individual hearing aid. This is especially helpful during the early stages of auditory training, to help you recognize the very fine distinctions between many sounds that are very similar. Once you have thoroughly absorbed these distinctions, you can carry them over into use with your own hearing aid. Sanders notes that "when we are attempting to learn a new activity, we require a great deal more information in learning to discriminate between sounds and words than we do to perform the same act of discrimination once we have learned these sound patterns."[3] If professional help is not available to you, you can still benefit from auditory training exercises with the help of a relative or friend. The suggestions in this chapter may also be used to *supplement* your clinical training. As J. C. Kelly points out, "the improvement of a perceptual skill usually requires an abundance of exercise rather than the limited amount provided in the clinical period."[4]

When should I begin auditory training practice? If you have a new hearing aid, it would be best to follow the suggestions in Chapter 8 for adjusting to the aid for a few weeks before you start the home practice exercises that follow. This doesn't mean that you must be completely adjusted to hearing aid use, but you should have at least arrived at some kind of acceptance of the aid under relatively unpressured conditions before you attempt auditory training at home.

Do I need a special place for auditory training practice? Best results are obtained in a room where room noise, echo, and distraction are kept to a minimum. This means, if possible, a carpeted room with closed drapes. This kind of environment cuts down on reverberation (sound bouncing off hard surfaces) and keeps outdoor sounds out as much as possible. If you're working in a large room, it will help to choose a corner that's as far away from the windows as possible and to place some high-backed chairs or a portable room divider screen nearby, draped with blankets.

Which should come first—auditory training or lipreading? Actually, as I mentioned in Chapter 9, the two skills should be combined during most of your practice sessions. The aim of both is to improve your ability to communicate, and the best way to do this is by using *all* of your senses to the fullest. I have divided my discussion of lipreading and auditory training into two chapters for convenience, but both of them should be part of your total aural rehabilitation program. If you receive professional help from an audiologist or speech and hearing clinic, your therapy sessions will include auditory training, lipreading, and speech training. These areas overlap and will often be combined. The same should be true of your practice sessions at home. You'll notice that I've made suggestions for combining these skills in Chapters 9, 10, and 11.

Are there any special requirements for the person who will be my at-home helper? First of all, he should know as much about your hearing problem as possible. If the helper is your husband or wife, your spouse should go with you to the otologist, audiologist, and hearing aid dealer. These people will familiarize him with the nature and extent of your problem and explain to him how your hearing aid works. If you are receiving help from a speech and hearing clinician, that person will tell your mate how he can help you at home to reinforce what is being done for you in the therapy sessions. It's also important that your helper have good, clear speech. Even though you can practice lipreading with a hard-of-hearing friend, it would not be advisable for you to work on auditory training with a hearing-impaired helper unless his speech is good.

How should I set my hearing aid for auditory-training practice at home? In the early stages, the volume control should be set at the level of loudness that is most comfortable for you. Later, you'll want to try to increase your tolerance for loudness. This is important for you if you have a problem with recruitment, or if your hearing aid bothers you simply because you're used to having all sounds softened by your hearing loss. If loud sounds bother you unduly, your hearing aid may be more of an annoyance than a help to you at first. You could decide it's nothing but a nuisance and relegate it to the dresser drawer. But there's a better solution. Kelly points out that "it has been demonstrated by the Harvard Psycho-acoustic Laboratory that the tender ear may be toughened after exposure to loud sounds. The tolerance levels may be improved considerably through reasonably short periods of exposure to amplified sound. Acceptance of greater intensity is one of the expected improvements in hearing aid use."[5] Still, you're never going to develop this "expected improvement" as long as your aid sits in the drawer. So get it out, put it on, and let's begin.

Increasing your tolerance for loudness is something that should be done gradually, a little bit at a time, as you proceed through the exercises in this chapter. I'm discussing it separately only to avoid repeating myself at each step throughout the chapter. (Have you ever tried to organize a book without losing your sanity???) Have your hearing aid set at the most comfortable level of loudness for the first few sessions. Then, choose a day when you're feeling relaxed, and have your helper read from a book or magazine in his normal voice as you adjust the volume control on your hearing aid. When you find the loudness level that is most comfortable for you, turn the volume up very slightly and continue with the auditory training lesson you're working on. Set your control at this new level for the next few sessions. You'll soon find that it is no longer unpleasantly loud. When you reach this point, turn it up again, very slightly, and keep it that way for the next few sessions. Continue increasing the loudness in very gradual steps, and you'll soon find that you can be comfortable with a considerably higher level of loudness than you could when you first started wearing your hearing aid. Remember, you'll be doing this tolerance work *while* you're working on the lessons in the rest of this chapter.

O K, so how do I begin with my auditory training? First, read this whole chapter through before you start your at-home practice. This will help you to get an overall view of where you're going, and it will give you some understanding of the principles involved. As in all learning tasks, it's best to begin with the simple things and work up gradually to the more complex. So it's important that you do the exercises in the order in which they are presented in the following pages. If the first few exercises are very easy for you, go right on until you come to a lesson in which you begin making mistakes. Then continue repeating the exercises suggested at that stage until you are satisfied with your ability to perform them. Don't expect perfection. Just keep at it until you feel you're doing as well as you can. If you reach a point at which you feel frustrated and discouraged, don't go on to harder lessons. Go back a lesson or two and practice that stage some more. You may be able to work up later.

If your hearing loss is severe, you'll want to begin with practice in identifying sounds other than speech sounds. Have your helper gather several household items that make characteristic sounds, such as a spoon stirring in a cup, keys jangling, a newspaper rattling, a handful of coins clinking, etc. Try to identify the source of each sound without looking. If you have no trouble doing this, proceed to discriminating among sounds that are more similar. Have your helper use various household items to make noises that are paired to sound rather similar. For instance, he can make a stirring noise with a

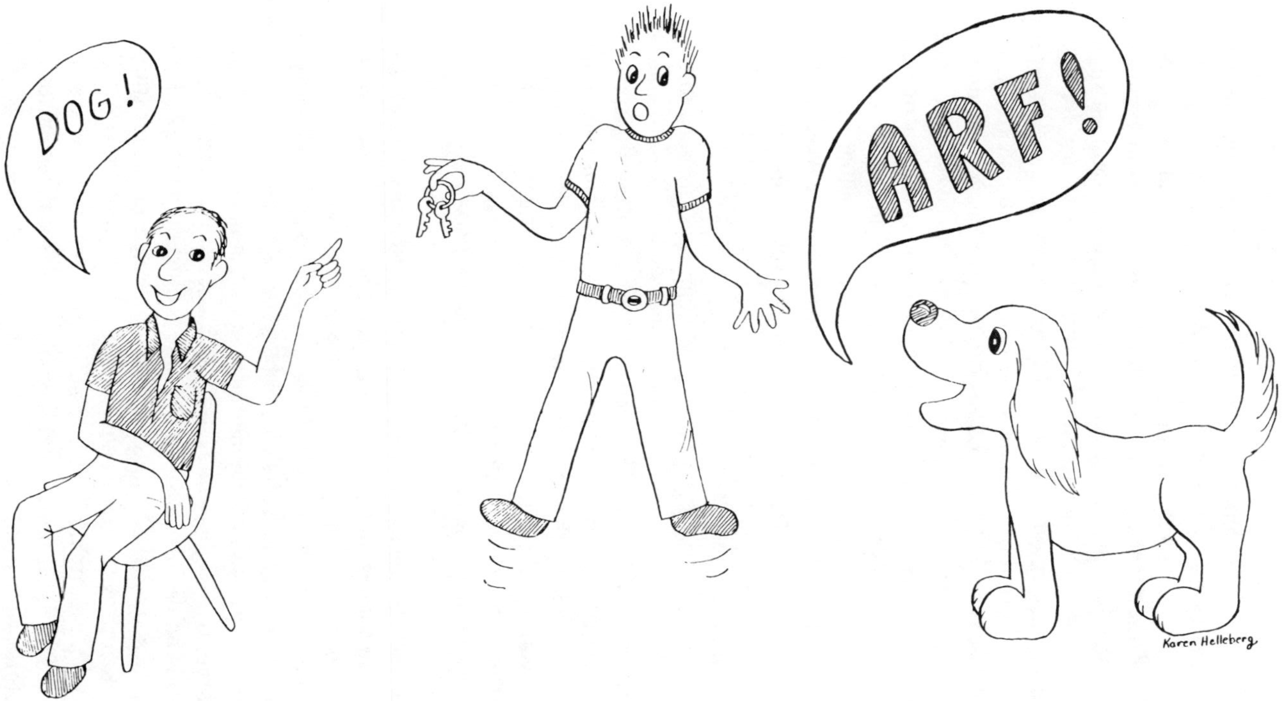

Figure 10.2. One good household sound deserves another!

spoon, first in a plastic cup, then in a glass dish, and then in a saucepan, while you try to identify which combination he's using. Or you can try to distinguish between the sound of running water and the sound of the TV turned to a channel that is not on the air, or between the sound of the front door closing and a cupboard door banging. Practice of this kind will help you to focus your attention on slight differences between similar sounds. If this seems too easy for you, your hearing loss is probably not severe enough to require gross sound discrimination practice. If so, go right on to the next lesson.

What is the next step? When you're able to easily distinguish among various sounds in your environment, you're ready to go on to practice in speech discrimination. The following suggestions for practice are based on the sequence presented by J. C. Kelly in his *Clinician's Handbook for Auditory Training.* This is a useful manual that contains specific directions for auditory training lessons as well as practice lists and answer sheets. You may want to order it from the Alexander Graham Bell Association for the Deaf, Inc., 3417 Volta Place, N. W., Washington, DC 20007.

A good way to begin is by using the numbers from zero to ten, because, with the exception of five and nine, each of these numbers has a different vowel sound. Sit the same distance from the speaker each time so that improvement can be noted under constant conditions. Face *away from* the speaker so that you won't be able to read his lips as you are listening. Now, take a lined sheet of paper and number from zero to ten vertically down the page. Have your helper call off various *pairs* of numbers, such as two, six—three, four—eight, one—four, nine—five, zero. He should say each digit separately (e.g., two, six—not twenty-six), and *0* should be called "zero," not "oh." He should always begin with the phrase, "Number one is . . ." or "Number two is . . .", etc. The speaker should write down the sequence he uses so that you can check your responses later. If you find it easy to recognize pairs of numbers, increase the difficulty by having your helper call off the numbers in sequences of three digits, such as three, five, eight—nine, zero, four—seven, two, six—etc. As soon as you can do this satisfactorily, add a fourth digit. Next, Kelly suggests proceeding to groupings of two numerals and a letter (three, eight, *t*), then three numerals and a letter (eight, four, *n,* seven).

Should I keep practicing on this lesson until I get all of the answers right? No. This is an unreasonable goal. As Kelly states, "with the history of hearing inaccuracy that most hard-of-hearing persons have, perfection is probably out of the question."[6] So stick with it until it becomes fairly easy for you, but not long enough to get bored or unduly frustrated. Then move on to the next lesson.

What comes next? When you find that you can discriminate among the numbers without too much trouble, follow the same procedure with the letters of the alphabet. Have your helper call off single letters (not in alphabetical order, of course) while you write them down. Again, this should first be done without watching the speaker's lips. Then check to see which ones you missed.

Since there are several letters that may sound alike to you, you'll probably find that you have made a number of errors. For instance, you may have written down *b* instead of *p,* or *m* instead of *n*. Now practice on those error sounds by having your helper pronounce them in pairs, pairing the sound he actually said with the one you wrote down. For instance, if he said *t* and you wrote down *d,* he should pair these two sounds (*d, t—t, d—t, d—d, t*—etc.) while you try to become aware of the very slight differences between the two sounds. This time, combine lipreading practice with your auditory training by watching his lips while he pronounces the letters.

Next, proceed to practice on three-letter series (*a, y, g—s, b, t—v, m, p*—etc.) Your helper should pause slightly between letters and not run them together. When you attain a reasonable measure of success with this, have your helper add a fourth letter to each grouping (*a, v, j, z—g, n, h, t—p, f, a, o*—etc.). You'll find this more difficult because it involves auditory memory, which is a faculty that may have fallen off for you since you've had your hearing loss. You'll get it back, though, with regular practice. When you're satisfied with your ability to do this (remember not to expect perfection), you're ready to move on to the next stage of auditory training.

What comes next? Now you can begin word discrimination practice. Have your helper pronounce one-syllable words in pairs (*house—boy;* not *wonder—heaven),* and then you repeat them. Doing it orally instead of on paper will save time. Try it first without watching his lips. When you make a mistake, have him write that pair of words down and later go back and pronounce them again. This time, watch his lips as he says the words. After he has pronounced, say, twenty pairs, he should go back and repeat the ones you missed. Practice on pairs of words until you feel fairly confident, and then go on to groups of three words, following the same procedure. Now the speaker should not pause between words. That way, the rhythm will be more nearly like that of conversational speech. If you have difficulty in identifying the words in this triple-word practice, ask your helper to prolong the vowel sound in the words (keeeeep). When you are able to correctly identify a reasonable percentage of three-series words, have your speaker pronounce four words at a time before you repeat them. When you first start practicing on this lesson, the words (still having only one syllable) may be chosen at random. Later, to increase the difficulty and give you practice in finer discrimination, your speaker should include in each group of four words some words that rhyme. Examples might be groupings such as these: *house,* boy, friend, *mouse—best, chest,* dirt, *messed—late,* care, *bait, date.* Notice that, in each grouping, there are two or more words that have the same vowel sound and end with the same consonant sound. This kind of practice forces you to discriminate between the words solely on the basis of the beginning consonant sounds, since the other sounds are alike. For this exercise, your helper will probably need to prepare his list ahead of time. If he has trouble thinking of enough one-syllable words that rhyme, he may want to consult a rhyming dictionary. Your library probably has one, or one can be purchased at a small cost in paperback at almost any bookstore.

What do I do after I have become fairly successful in identifying these four-word groups? When you have reached this point, your discrimination ability for words should be quite good. Now you are ready to have your helper present you with short sentences of no more than five or six words, such as: *The dog wants in. Today is Friday, February twentieth. It is time to eat now.* As before, repeat the sentences after him. For variation, he may ask you short questions. Instead of repeating these, give him an answer that will show him that you understood the question. You'll probably find this sentence practice easier than identifying groups of four unrelated words. This is because the context, or sense, of the sentence helps you. In fact, I'm betting you'll whiz through this practice on short sentences. If so, your speaker can increase the sentence length. Then he can talk to you using two or three sentences at a time. Now, instead of trying to repeat what he says word for word, just tell him in your own words what you think he has said.

Next, your helper can read a paragraph to you from a magazine or book, making sure first that you know the subject of the article or chapter so you'll have something to go on. When he has finished reading the paragraph, see if you can tell him, in your own words, what it said.

Once I can understand sentences in sequence, am I through with auditory training? There's another step that will help you to get along better in difficult listening situations, such as at parties, in restaurants and airports, etc. Oh, I know, you're probably tired of this kind of work by now (and I *know* it's work, believe me), but if you've come this close to breaking that sound barrier, why not rev up your mental engines and push on through?

Many situations you'll encounter in everyday life will require understanding of speech under less-than-ideal conditions. You'll need practice in mentally separating the speech message you're trying to understand from distracting background noise. As Sanders points out, this ability is largely psychological, and with practice, "a subject can learn to improve speech discrimination under these conditions."[7] The beginning user of a hearing aid is in somewhat the same situation as a student pilot who is learning to use his radio for communication. When I first started my flying lessons, I had a terrible time understanding those voices coming over the radio from the control tower. There was a great deal of static, interference, and distortion. Through practice, though, I gradually learned to ignore the static and the other pilots' voices that interfered and to give my complete listening attention to that one voice that was directing me. When you're wearing your hearing aid in a noisy place, you may at first hear nothing but "garble." If you'll practice at home, listening to your helper in the presence of background noise, you'll soon learn to mentally shut out the distraction and attend only to the speaker. Then going out among people will be easier for you.

How do I provide this background noise? There are several ways. You can turn on the radio or television. You can use a record player or tape recorder. I've found that the best way to begin this phase is by using music, because it is obviously not as distracting as speech. Sit facing your helper, with the distraction noise off to one side. Do not try to get the message without watching his lips. You'll need all the help you can get for this exercise! Your helper should speak in sentences for this practice. Do not try to repeat his message word for word. Concentrate on getting the gist of what he says. Start with a comfortable volume setting on your hearing aid, and set the volume of the background noise rather low. Later, you can build up the noise to speech ratio by increasing the background noise. Next, if you have a tape recorder, take it to a very noisy place, such as a busy city street corner, and record the sounds of traffic. If you have a record player but not a tape recorder, you can buy a sound-effects record for this purpose. When you have completed several sessions using nonspeech background noises, move on to distractions composed of speech. A radio or TV newscast would be good for this, or an interview program or talk show. Again, begin with a low volume setting for the background noise, and work up until the distraction becomes almost as loud as your helper's voice. Keep these sessions short, and don't allow yourself to get discouraged. Listening situations of this kind are difficult even for people with normal hearing. But if you'll stick with it, you'll soon find that your growing ability to separate irrelevant sounds from what you *want* to hear will carry over into your everyday life.

I asked you in the beginning of this chapter to read all the way through it before starting your auditory training. Now you are ready to go back and begin the lessons. At this point, if it's your first reading, you may be somewhat doubtful about the value of all this practice. All I can tell you is that auditory training has helped many others who have had problems similar to yours. Why settle for less than the best your ears can do for you?

11

What can I do to keep my hearing and my speech from getting worse?

At the beginning of Chapter 1, I told you about the coins I lost on my way to the store to buy a kite. If I had discovered at any point along my route to the store that some of the coins were missing, what do you think I would have done? Right! I would have snapped my purse shut *right then,* to keep from losing any more. There are things *you* can do, at the first sign of hearing loss, to protect your remaining hearing. True, some hearing losses are progressive and will get worse no matter what you do. But even if you have a progressive type of loss, you'll want to take every possible precaution to avoid *speeding up* the progression. The very fact that you have a hearing problem may mean that your ears are unusually susceptible to damage from such things as infection, ototoxic drugs (*oto*, "ear"; *toxic*, "physically damaging"), allergy, or noise. In addition to protecting your remaining hearing, you'll also want to do everything you can to keep your speech from deteriorating. Let's talk about the hearing part first.

How often should I have my hearing retested? By all means, have your hearing rechecked periodically—at *least* once a year and more frequently if your hearing specialist recommends it *or* if you notice a change in your hearing ability. *Always* have your hearing tested after you've had an upper respiratory infection or a severe bout with an allergy. If head noise, or tinnitus, increases, it's time for a recheck regardless of how long it's been since you had it done.

How can my family physician help? He can immunize you against many of the infectious diseases that damage hearing. You should seriously consider having flu shots, particularly when there is an impending epidemic of the respiratory type of influenza. You should also ask your doctor to check your ears periodically for wax buildup. Of course, it goes without saying that, for you, the slightest earache, or even an uncomfortable feeling of fullness in the ears, demands immediate medical attention. A head cold that seems to "settle in the ears" should never be left to run its course.

What can other specialists do to help me save the hearing I have left? If allergies are a problem for you, make an appointment with an allergist. He may put you on a program of desensitizing shots and/or prescribe antihistamine medication. Allergy can add to your hearing impairment even if it isn't the main cause of your problem. Don't take a chance on that.

Keep your teeth in good condition by regular visits to the dentist. If you let them decay to the point that extractions are necessary, your bite may be affected. If your jaws get too far out of alignment, their position could partially or completely close off your ear canal, *increasing* your hearing problem.

What about medications? You should avoid taking aspirin if possible, since some people are susceptible to ear damage from it. There are nonprescription pain relievers on the market now that don't contain any aspirin. Never take streptomycin, neomycin, or kanamycin unless your life is at stake. When your doctor prescribes *any* antibiotic, always ask him if it has been thoroughly tested for possible ototoxic effects.

Must I stop smoking? As I mentioned in a previous chapter, there is some evidence that smoking may cause hearing damage in some people. More research needs to be done in this area. Still, if there's a chance that smoking may add to your hearing defect, it would certainly seem worthwhile to stop smoking, or at least cut down, if you're a heavy smoker.

The same may be said for drinking large amounts of coffee or tea. I'd recommend cutting out or down on these beverages, at least for a period of several months, to see if abstaining from them slows down the progression of your hearing loss.

Will wearing my hearing aid regularly help conserve my hearing? Well, not in the sense that it would *improve* your hearing acuity or stop a progressive loss. It won't do either of these things. But, if you wear it regularly, it may very well *conserve your ability to understand* what you hear. Understanding speech is a *learned* skill that develops from listening practice. The ability to discriminate among speech sounds deteriorates rapidly when a hearing loss sets in. At the risk of oversimplifying, let's say that, if you wear your hearing aid regularly, you can keep the "brain connections" that are used for interpreting speech active so they won't get "rusty." In this way, regular wearing of your hearing aid will help you to protect the *usability* of the hearing you have left.

What is the greatest environmental threat to my hearing? *Noise* wins that one, hands down. Our world is becoming increasingly noisy, to the point that it's almost impossible to live in it without being exposed, at least part of the time, to potentially damaging noise. Some experts have even suggested that the loss of hearing that occurs with aging may be largely due to the everyday assault of environmental noises on our hearing mechanism. "There is evidence to suggest that primitive tribesmen in Africa who are completely removed from the noise of our modern civilization do not show any appreciable decrease in hearing acuity with advancing age."[1]

The worst thing about noise-induced hearing loss is that it usually happens so gradually that the person is not aware of any change in his hearing until the damage has become permanent.

Why is this? There are two reasons. First, noise doesn't usually cause discomfort until it reaches a level of about 120 decibels, so you could work all day in noise of 90–100 decibels without being terribly uncomfortable. You might notice some ringing in the ears or muffling of sound at the end of the day or at the end of the week, but the problem would go away after a good night's sleep or a weekend away from the noise. If you had your hearing tested at the end of the work day on Friday, your audiogram might show a slight loss, but a retest on Monday morning would probably show that your hearing had returned to normal. This is called *temporary threshold shift,* and it's easy to shrug off as a minor annoyance. *But,* after several weeks or months (depending on how sensitive your ears are to noise), the loss would begin to show up on the Monday morning audiogram, too. It wouldn't be as great as Friday's loss, but it would increase gradually as time went on.

The second reason you probably wouldn't notice the damage until it was too late is that, in noise-induced hearing loss, the higher frequencies are affected first. A slight high-frequency loss doesn't interfere much with your understanding of speech, so you wouldn't notice the change. If noise exposure continues, though, the loss will gradually "bleed over" into the middle frequencies. When this happens, you'll begin to suspect that you're not hearing as well as you used to. By this time, the loss may have become permanent.

If I have a noise-induced loss, will my hearing return to normal if I change to a job in quieter surroundings? It may, over a period of several weeks or months, if the problem is discovered early enough and the change is made immediately. On the other hand, it may not. Either way, changing to a quieter job can prevent further loss of hearing. If you work in a noisy factory, or operate noise-producing farm machinery, or pilot a plane, or do anything else that exposes you to excessive levels of noise, you'd better *do something* about it. This is especially true if you already have a hearing loss, regardless of the cause. I'll discuss ear protection in a minute.

But won't I just get used to the racket after a while? *No!* Or, let me revise that: if you think you're getting used to the noise, it's probably because your hearing has deteriorated. "If, after long exposure to noise, you stop hearing it, it's because you've become *deaf*."[2]

Must I quit my job? This is a decision only you can make. It might be the wisest thing to do. Or maybe your company can place you in a position where the noise levels are not so great. If you do continue to work in noisy surroundings, by all means use ear protectors.

What kind of ear protectors should I use? Two basic types are available: ear plugs that are inserted into the ear canal, and earmuffs that fit over the entire outer ear.

If you choose the insert type, don't just go to the store and buy a set of ear plugs, such as those used for swimming. In order to be effective against noise, ear plugs must fit tightly in the ear canal so that no air can get through. You may need one size for one ear and another size for the other ear. They should be fitted by a trained person. Your audiologist may do this for you, or some hearing-aid dealers can fit you with custom-molded ear plugs that are just right for you. The dealer casts a mold of your ear, sends it to his company, and they send you a soft rubber insert that matches the mold. These should be used by adults only, because children's and teenagers' ear canal shapes change rapidly, and protection may become inadequate in a few months.

Over-the-ear muffs can provide a somewhat better level of sound reduction than inserts can. And if you have a draining ear or a chronic infection, plug inserts may aggravate the condition. In this case, you should definitely use muff-type protectors. Also, some people have ear canals that simply do not accept ear-plug insertion without discomfort. If you have this problem, earmuffs are the best choice for you. They completely cover the ears, and a tensioned headband holds them snugly in place. The cups of the headmuffs should be made of sponge in the area where they contact the head so that a good seal is formed. Be sure to push your hair out of the way when putting the

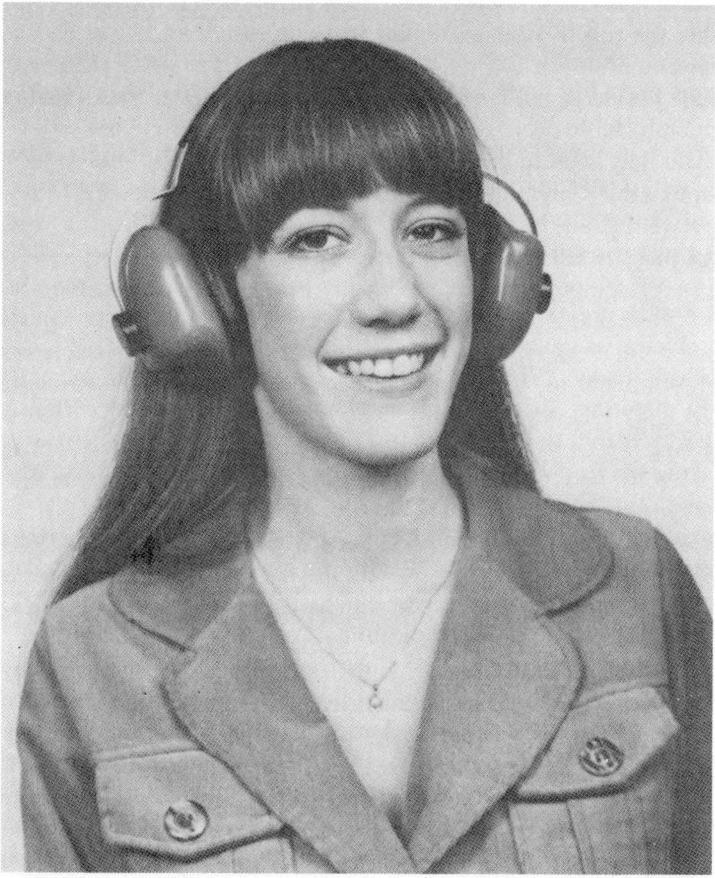

Figure 11.1. Muff-type ear protectors give valuable protection against damaging noise.

muffs on, so it won't interfere with this seal. Muff-type protectors cost more than inserts to begin with but may save you money in the long run, because ear plugs are easily lost, and you may have to replace them several times. Some people feel that the muffs are more comfortable for daily use than the inserts.

On the other hand, if you wear glasses, muffs may not work for you, because the bows of your glasses may interfere with the ability of the muff to seal off incoming sound. If you work in a hot room or out in the sun in the summertime, earmuffs may be uncomfortable for you.

You should use whatever type of ear protection is the most comfortable for you in your particular working situation. If you choose the most comfortable device, you'll be more likely to wear it throughout your period of noise exposure, and that's far better than wearing an uncomfortable device only part of the time. For maximum protection, you may want to use *both* ear plugs and earmuffs. Studies have shown that this combination provides the greatest amount of attenuation, or reduction, in sound level.

Can't I just use cotton to plug my ears? Dry cotton is almost useless as an ear protector, and it creates its own problems in that people who use it *believe* that their ears are protected; so they continue to expose themselves to damaging noise. There *are* some types of disposable ear protectors made of wax-impregnated cotton, or of other specially treated materials, that are reasonably effective, but plain cotton is *not.* Using cotton to keep noise out of your ears is about as effective as making the roof of your house out of screening and expecting it to keep the rain out!

But won't ear protectors make it hard for me to hear instructions and warnings? Surprisingly, no. With the distracting noise cut down, you'll be able to hear speech and signals better than when the background noise was masking them out.[3]

Will I have to give up hunting? It isn't surprising that many hunters and servicemen have noise-induced hearing losses, when you consider the high-intensity noise produced by gunshot plus the blast impact of this close-to-the-ear noise. In right-handed people, the damage is likely to be greater in the left ear, which they point toward the muzzle. The reverse is true for left-handers. *Never* fire a gun without wearing ear protectors, no matter what the caliber. And insist that observers wear ear protection, too, when you're shooting.

Shooting creates some special problems in ear protection. Walter Leonetti has pointed out in an article for *The American Rifleman:*

> The highest portion of the lower jaw borders on the floor of the ear canal. Every time you place a stock against your cheek, you run the risk of breaking the seal of the ear protector. The better fitting the stock, the less risk. A good rule to follow is to test for the seal then check your stock. Rather than fire, re-check the seal by smacking two pieces of metal together. The sound should be muffled. If it is not, your ears are not protected. The checking process sounds involved but should take no longer than five seconds. Chewing gum or yawning can also break a seal.[4]

There is a third type of ear protector that may be used to cushion you against impact noise, such as that of a gun firing, but this type is not useful for constant noise. It's the piston-type ear plug, which allows sound to proceed normally through the ear canal until a blast occurs. Then the sound waves force the plug inward long enough to seal off the opening during the duration of the blast.

How loud does noise have to be to damage my hearing? This is a hard question to answer because the results of noise exposure depend on several factors, including overall loudness, frequency range, the number of hours of exposure each day, and the number of years of continued exposure. Then, as I've said before, individuals vary in their susceptibility to noise-induced hearing loss.

In 1970, the Occupational Safety and Health Act (OSHA) was passed in the United States, limiting the levels of allowable noise in factories that have federal contracts and in all manufacturing plants engaging in interstate commerce. Table 11.1 shows the levels of daily noise exposure permissible under this act. Some experts feel that these levels are still too high to be considered safe, and they suggest that the maximum allowable noise for an eight-hour working day should be under eighty decibels.[5]

Table 11.1
Allowable daily noise exposures according to
Occupational Safety and Health Act

Duration per day, hours	Sound level, decibels
8	90
6	92
4	95
3	97
2	100
1½	102
1	105
½	110
¼ or less	115

From Department of Labor, Occupational Safety and Health Administration, "Occupational Safety and Health Standards" in *Federal Register* Vol. 37 No. 202 Part II, p. 22157.

How loud is eighty decibels? To give you some basis for comparison, here are some common noise levels, with their loudness given in decibels:

jet plane (140)
gunshot blast (140)
automobile horn (120)
woodworking shop (100)

boiler shop (100)
subway (90)
average factory (80–90)
noisy restaurant (80)
busy traffic (75)
conversational speech (66)
average home (50)
soft whisper (30).[6]

An increase of only ten decibels on a PNdB (perceived noise decibel) scale means that the noise has *doubled* in intensity.

If no sound-measuring devices are available, how do I know if I need protection? A good rule of thumb is this: If you have to raise your voice to be heard by someone less than two feet away, you should be wearing a protective device.[7] If your job exposes you to noises that are this loud, you should have your hearing checked as often as once a week if possible. If such frequent testing is not feasible, you should definitely wear ear protectors or find other employment.

What about environmental noise over which I have no control? If you live in a large metropolitan area, or near an airport where jets take off and land regularly, you may be exposed to damaging noise beyond your control. David Lipscomb has noted that "noise levels in numerous cities have increased 20 decibels in the past 20 years."[8] What can you do? You can dampen the amount of noise that reaches you inside your home by keeping your windows closed, putting up heavy, porous drapes, installing acoustical-tile ceilings, and carpeting your floors. You should do everything in your power to persuade your local government to pass and enforce reasonable noise regulations. In many areas, citizens' groups have been formed for this purpose. The public is becoming increasingly aware of the damaging effects of noise, and those in power are beginning to listen. Let's hope that, in the near future, our knowledge of technology will be put to use to reduce the noise levels of trucks, construction equipment, jet aircraft, farming equipment, and other noisemakers that may be chiseling away at our hearing ability. Write letters. Get on the phone. Stir up your neighbors. People in power have ears, too. *Make* them listen. Stop *ear* pollution.

Can loud rock 'n' roll music cause hearing damage? A considerable amount of research has been done on this question in the past few years, and the results of the studies do not always agree. It has been established that exposure to rock 'n' roll music produces at least a temporary threshold shift. Furthermore, average levels of rock 'n' roll music (104–111 dB) do fall in the damaging category, and musicians and others whose jobs expose them to this noise have a greater incidence of high-frequency hearing loss. On the other hand, according to William Rintelmann, most people "could probably tolerate one or two exposure periods per week for a few years with negligible risk of an educationally or socially significant hearing impairment."[9] Until conclusive answers to this question are found, common sense should direct you to stay away from excessive exposure to this high-powered music, especially if you already have a hearing loss. If you're a rock 'n' roll musician or an employee of a discotheque, better wear ear protectors. Insert-type protectors are practically unnoticeable, and they may save you from losing your ability to enjoy music of any kind!

The first half of this chapter has been concerned with hearing conservation. Now let's talk a little bit about *speech* conservation.

Why do I need to be concerned about my speech? Because the movements required for good speech are so intricate, and because the least change in the position of the tongue, lips, teeth, and other parts of the speech mechanism results in distortion of speech sounds, we need to be constantly making minor adjustments in order to keep our speech clear and precise. We make these adjustments *automatically* in response to the way our speech *sounds* to us as we talk. When our hearing becomes defective, we lose some of our ability to monitor our own speech, so our articulation begins to deteriorate. We also pattern our speech on the way *other people* sound to us. A hearing loss causes the speech of others to sound "mushy" and slurred to us and, after a while, we are speaking the way other people sound *to us*. Something similar to this happens when a person from Boston moves to Dallas. After he has lived in Texas for a while, he goes home for a visit and his friends tell him he has picked up a Southern accent. The more pronounced your hearing loss is, the greater the change it is likely to make in your speech patterns, but even a slight loss can cause speech problems. For instance, even a mild high-frequency hearing loss may cause the *s* and *z* sounds to lose their sharpness.

What if my hearing loss is only in one ear? Speech will probably not become a problem for you because your one good ear can still monitor your articulation, inflection, voice quality, and intensity. But there are several other factors that do determine a person's need for speech conservation or retraining.

How does age at the time of onset of hearing loss relate to speech?

Obviously, the child who is born deaf will learn to talk only if he has intensive speech and language training. On the other hand, the adult who loses his hearing, or part of it, has already developed language abilities, and his speech is likely to be adequate at the time the loss occurs. If he begins a program of speech conservation as soon as his hearing loss is discovered, he may be able to keep his speech from deteriorating. This is very important because, once defective speech patterns have taken over, it's difficult to correct them. To paraphrase Ben Franklin's adage, an ounce of speech conservation therapy is worth a pound of speech retraining. So if you have a significant hearing loss, particularly if it's a progressive one, find a good speech therapist at once. If you don't know of one in your area, write to American Speech and Hearing Association, 10801 Rockville Pike, Rockville, MD 20852. They'll direct you to a qualified clinician in your area.

But what if I still talk as well as I ever did? Are you *sure* you do? Sometimes the changes are so gradual that you are unaware of them. Even family members may not notice your speech deteriorating, since they are around you all the time. At any rate, it won't hurt to have an evaluation by a trained person. He may not recommend speech therapy at this time, but if not, he'll probably give you some suggestions to keep your speech from becoming impaired. You'll find some self-help suggestions at the end of this chapter, too.

Does a sudden loss hurt speech more than a gradual one? Usually it does. The adult who gradually loses more and more of his hearing makes continuing adjustments along the way, but the individual who wakes up one morning and finds himself deprived of his hearing can't do this. In either case, "the adjustment is helped considerably by persons who avail themselves of the necessary rehabilitative procedures: speech reading, auditory training, speech therapy, and speech conservation."[10]

How does my speech sound to others? Hearing loss can cause several types of defective speech, depending on the *type* and *degree* of the loss. There is almost always a problem with volume, or loudness. We use our hearing as a "thermostat" to control the intensity of our voices. As I explained in Chapter 3, if you have a conductive hearing loss, you're apt to speak too softly. If your problem is sensori-neural, you probably talk too loudly.

Another type of speech problem caused by hearing impairment is a defect of *quality*. You may not have trouble this way unless your hearing loss is severe. What happens is this: The severely hard-of-hearing person unconsciously feels the need to be aware of his voice production. Since he can't get this awareness through hearing, he tries to get it through the sense of touch. The sensation of touch is more acute toward the back of the throat than it is in the mouth, so he shifts his voice back there. This results in kind of a muffled, throaty voice that is often described as "deaf quality." People with conductive losses are apt to have a lack of nasal resonance. For instance, they tend to produce *m, n,* and *ng* as *b, d,* and *g* respectively, making their speech sound as if they had a head cold, while the individual with a sensori-neural loss is likely to have *too much* nasality.

Our ears also tell us to use rising and falling *inflections* to clarify the meaning of our words. This, too, is an automatic thing when our hearing is normal, but a significant hearing loss causes these inflections to flatten out, giving the voice a monotonous, lifeless quality.

One of the most noticeable changes hearing loss causes in speech is in the area of articulation. Your impaired hearing may be causing you to distort some sounds, to substitute one sound for another, and/or to omit certain sounds. If your problem is sensori-neural, your articulation may be severely affected, especially in the high frequency consonant sounds such as *s, z, ch, dj,* (as in *j*uice), *th, sh,* and *zh* (as in trea*s*ure). These sounds may become too "slushy" after your hearing has been impaired for a while. Eventually, if steps are not taken to conserve your speech, you may begin omitting them altogether without realizing that you're doing so.

So what can I do to keep my speech from deteriorating? Your best bet is to locate a speech and hearing clinician who has been specifically trained to help you. Programs of speech conservation or "speech insurance" are available in many communities to prevent speech defects from occurring in the hard-of-hearing population. The clinician will probably enlist the aid of one of the members of your family to help you with practice at home.

In case it is impossible for you to obtain professional speech therapy, here are some suggestions for you to follow to help you keep control of your speech.

First, use part of the practice time you have set aside for auditory training and lipreading. Remind yourself that, as Dr. Phillip Rosenberg points out, "speech defects associated with hearing losses may well be as handicapping and embarrassing as the hearing loss itself and every effort should be made to avoid or correct such defects."[11]

Ask your husband or wife or another family member who has normal hearing and normal speech to serve as your "second ear." As we discuss these suggestions, let's refer to this person as your family helper.

TO DEVELOP LOUDNESS CONTROL Raymond Carhart suggests practicing speaking at four or five levels of loudness, from very soft to very loud. Pay particular attention to the way each of these levels *feels* in your larynx (voice box) until you can tell, just by the sense of touch, at which of the four or five levels you are speaking. You will be able to judge this by the amount of pressure you feel in the vocal folds as you speak. Mentally number these loudness levels, from the softest (1) to the loudest (5). Practice until you can shift at will from one level to another. With the aid of your family helper, determine which of these levels is likely to be appropriate in various sound environments.[12] For instance, you can try out your four or five levels the next time you go out to a noisy restaurant. You and your family helper can decide which level of loudness is best in that situation. If it happens to be number four, you can make it a point to use the number four level of loudness whenever you're in a noisy restaurant. As you read this, the task may sound quite difficult, but with just a little practice, you'll find that you'll get the feel of it. It's a good idea to write down your classifications and carry the list in your billfold or purse so you can refer to it whenever necessary. Also, you should train yourself to notice the reactions of those around you. If they seem to be having trouble hearing you, *increase* your vocal *pressure* to the next level of loudness.

It's a little more difficult to judge when you are talking too loud. The best way to control this is to keep decreasing the intensity of your voice until people begin to show signs of difficulty in hearing you. Then increase to the next level of loudness and you should be just right.

TO IMPROVE YOUR VOICE QUALITY This is a bit more difficult. Newby has observed that pitch and intensity can be controlled through awareness of muscle position and movement, "but apparently vocal quality is almost entirely dependent on auditory monitoring."[13] If you have a hearing aid, you can ask your family helper to tell you when your voice quality sounds most natural, and then you can try to maintain that quality by listening to yourself as you speak. If you have a conductive loss and your voice is *lacking* in nasality, you can practice speaking with your fingers placed gently on the bony part of your nose. You should feel vibrations when you voice such sounds as *m, n,* and *ng.* If at first you don't feel vibration there, practice speaking lists of words having these three sounds until you consistently feel nasal resonance. If you have a sensori-neural loss resulting in *too much* nasality, practice speaking with your fingers placed on your nose and try to *eliminate* vibration there, except for the three nasal sounds.

TO OVERCOME VOCAL MONOTONY Practice reading sentences or paragraphs aloud while your family helper raises or lowers his finger to indicate the need for higher or lower pitch. Of course, the sentences you read are not the sentences you'll be using in conversations, but practice in varying your pitch will carry over into your everyday speech. If you practice regularly, you'll keep yourself conscious of the need for inflection, and your speech will remain more natural than it would be if you allowed it to flatten out into a mere drone.

TO CORRECT FAULTY ARTICULATION Here, a good hearing aid can be a great help to you. It may make it possible for you to *hear* some of the articulation errors in your own speech. Even if you don't wear your hearing aid at all times, do *always* wear it during your speech practice period. If you have professional help with speech retraining and conservation, your clinician will no doubt ask you to use an auditory training unit. Because this instrument is larger than a hearing aid, its earphones can provide greater amplification and less distortion than your own aid can. The training unit also has separate volume and tone controls for each ear. If your hearing aid or the auditory training unit can increase the amount of usable hearing available to you, you may be able to correct your articulation errors by this means. However, if your hearing loss is severe, you may need additional help from your other senses in overcoming your articulation problem.

Study the diagrams in Figures 11.2-11.17. They show how the speech organs should be positioned for each of the consonant sounds. Practice making each sound according to the diagrams, and ask your family helper to tell you when you are producing the sounds correctly. Then memorize the *feel* of the correct positions for the sounds you normally produce incorrectly. This is called *phonetic placement* and, though it is not as effective as auditory monitoring, it can be very useful to you in correcting faulty articulation. If your hearing loss is progressive, begin, while your speech is still good, to memorize the feel of correctly articulated sounds, particularly the *s, z, r, l, sh,* and *ch* sounds. These are the sounds that are most likely to deteriorate as your hearing loss worsens. For instance, if you know how a good, sharp *s* sound should *feel* when you say it, you can make a conscious effort to produce it correctly, even when you can no longer hear that

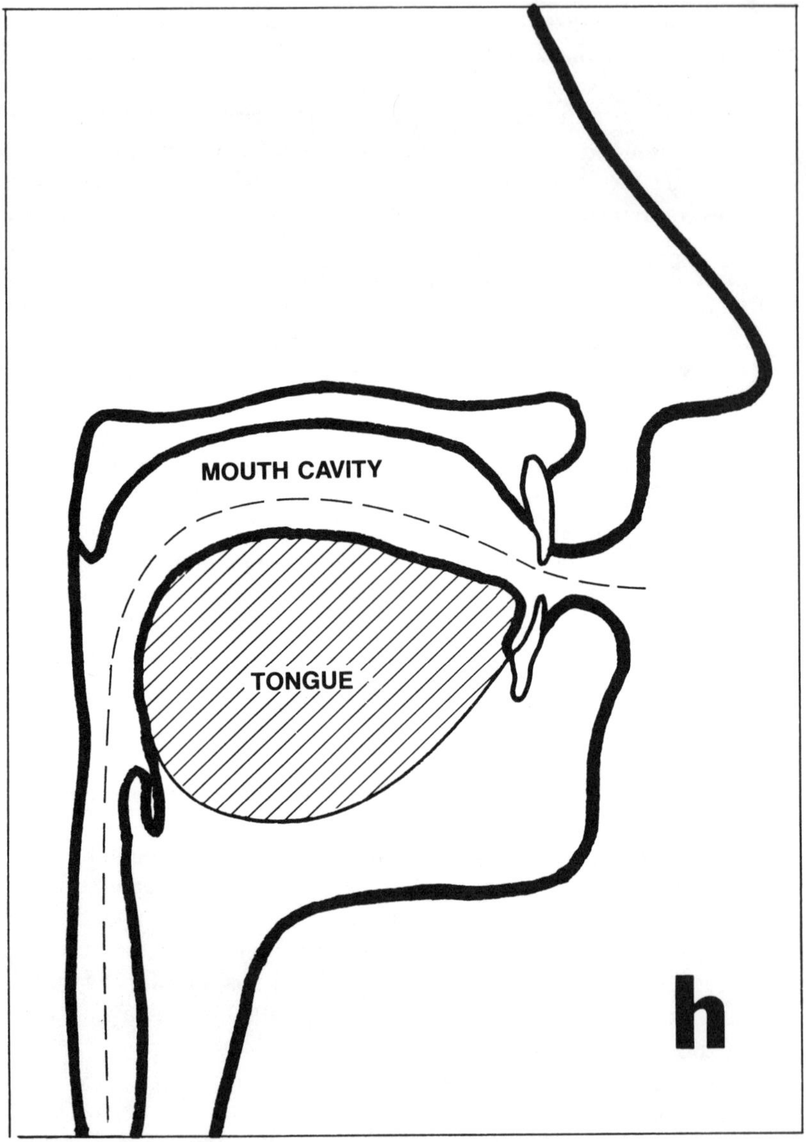

Figure 11.2. *h:* Tongue is in a relaxed position; mouth is slightly open; breath is exhaled forcefully.

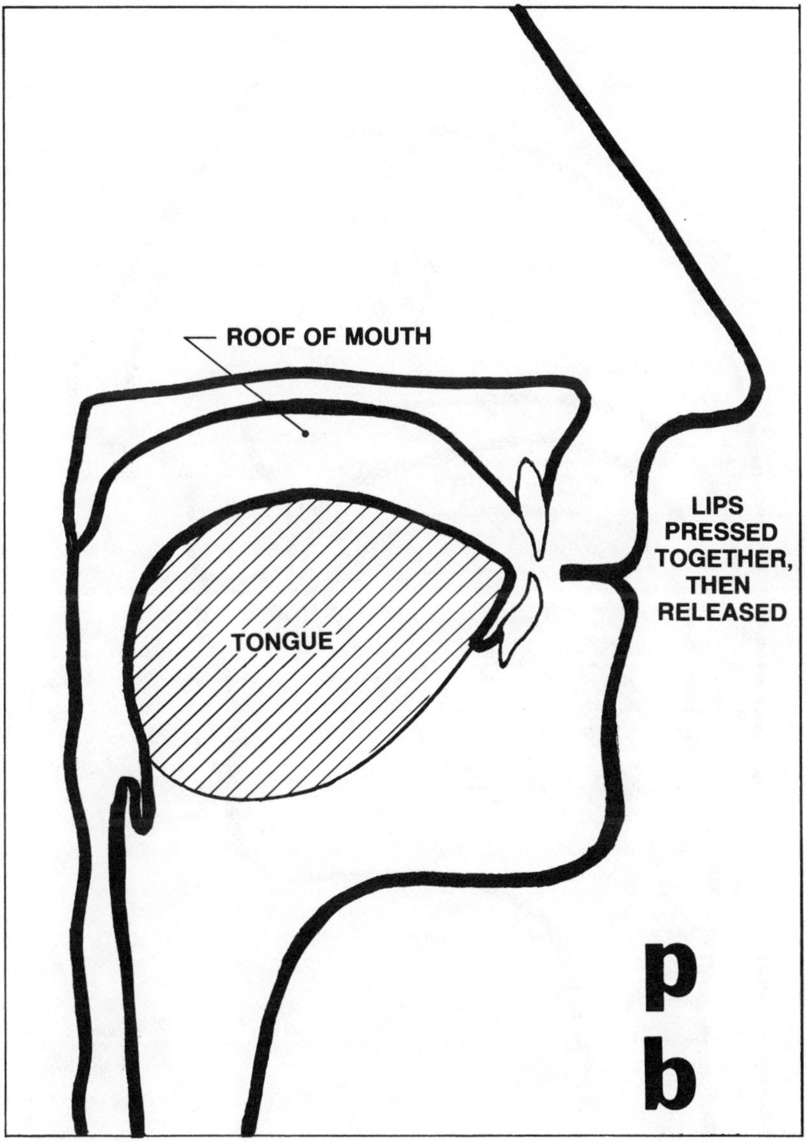

Figure 11.3. *p, b:* Tongue is relaxed; lips are pressed together, then released sharply; *p* is produced without voice; *b* is voiced.

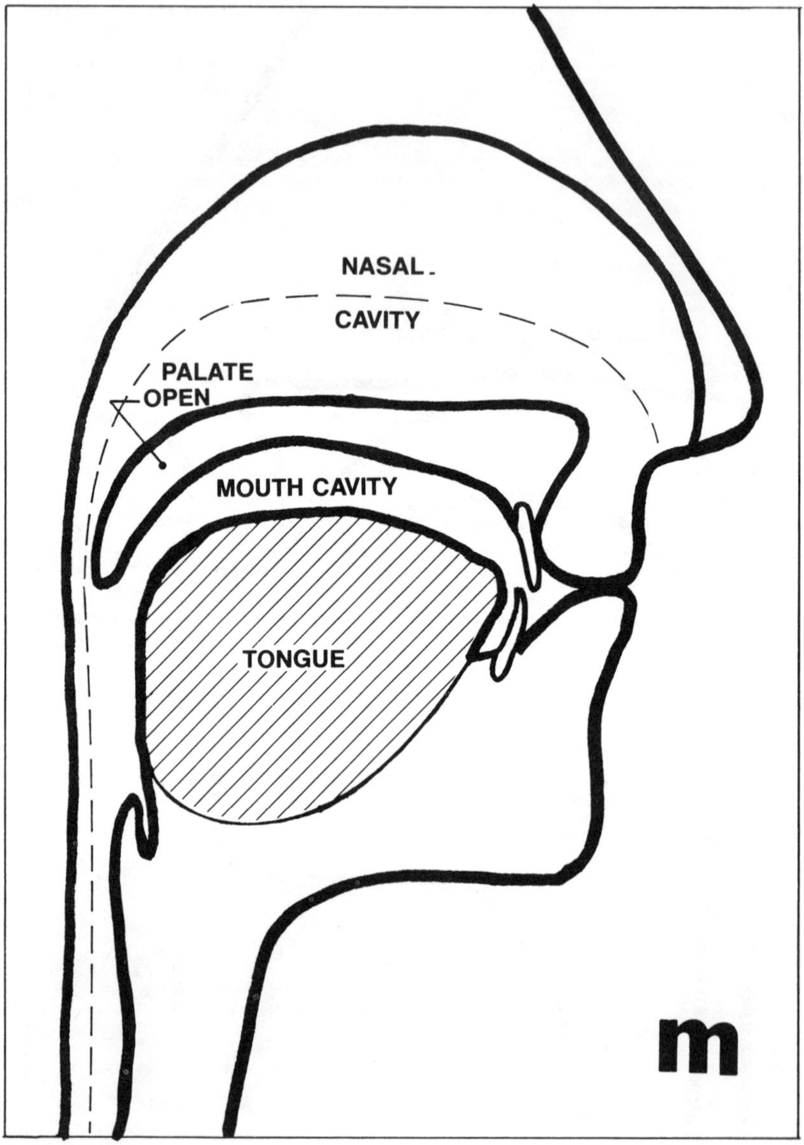

Figure 11.4. *m:* Lips are closed; soft palate is open so that voiced breath passes out through nose.

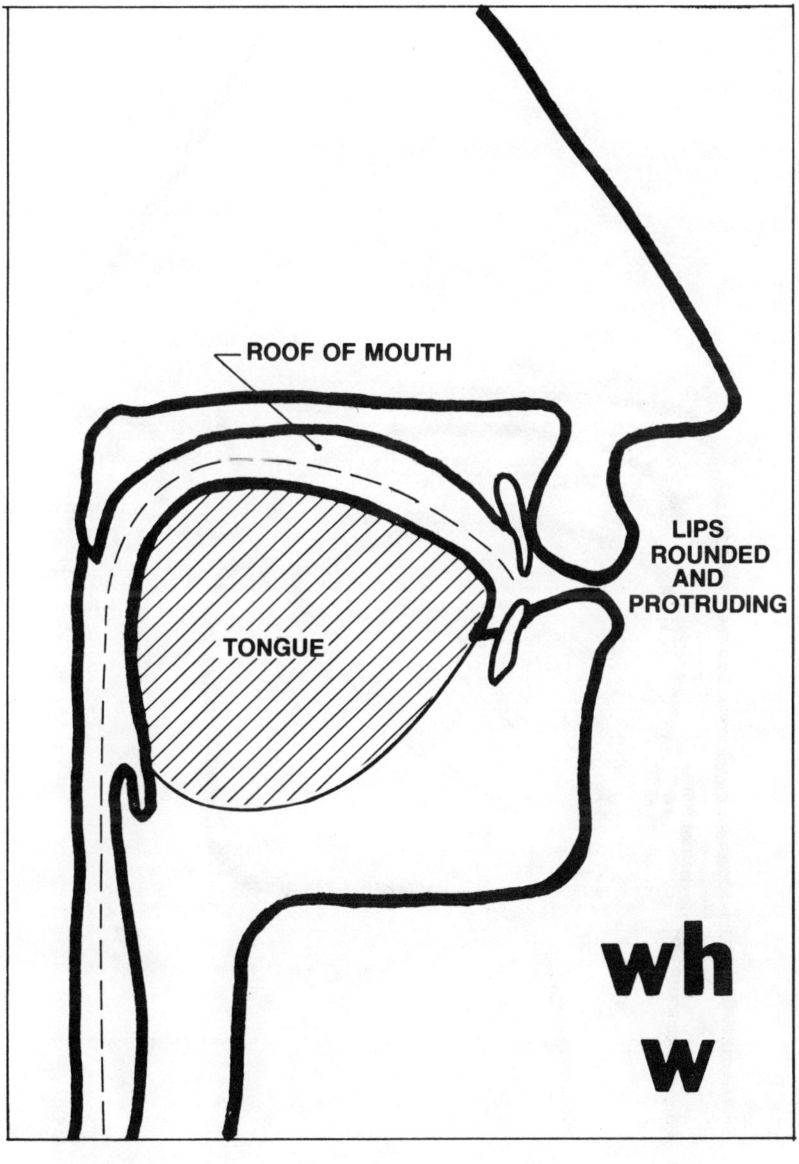

Figure 11.5. *wh, w:* Lips are rounded and protruding; back of tongue is raised slightly; *wh* is produced with greater force of air movement than for *w*.

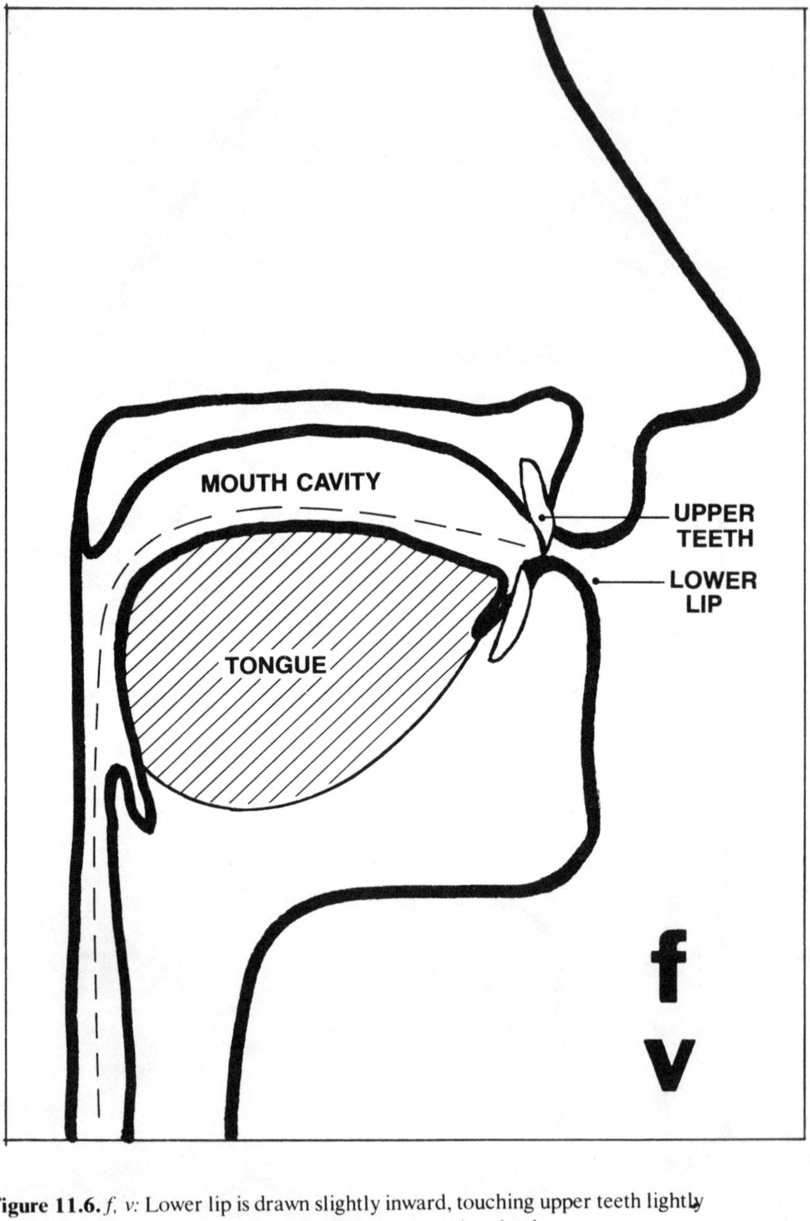

Figure 11.6. *f, v:* Lower lip is drawn slightly inward, touching upper teeth lightly enough for airstream to pass through; *f* is voiceless; *v* is voiced.

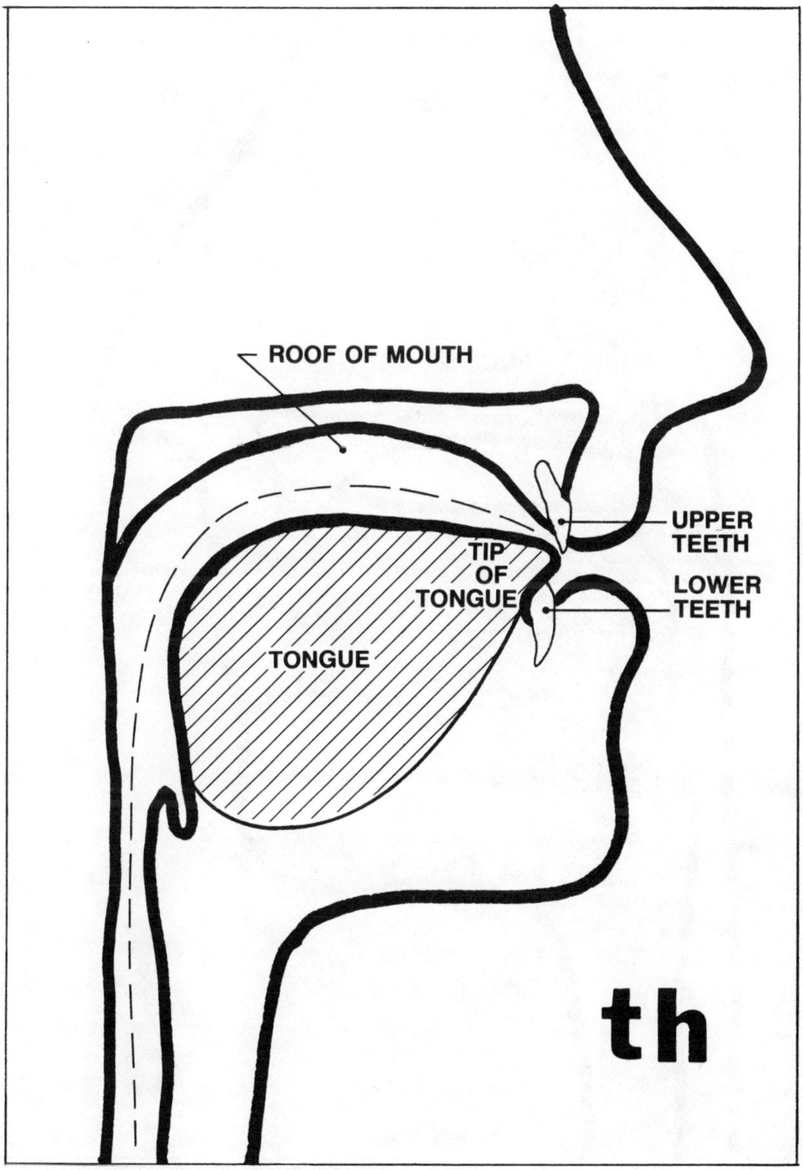

Figure 11.7. *th:* Tip of tongue, flattened, is placed against upper teeth, lightly enough for airstream to pass through; some *th* sounds are voiced (as in *th*ese), while some are voiceless (as in *th*ree).

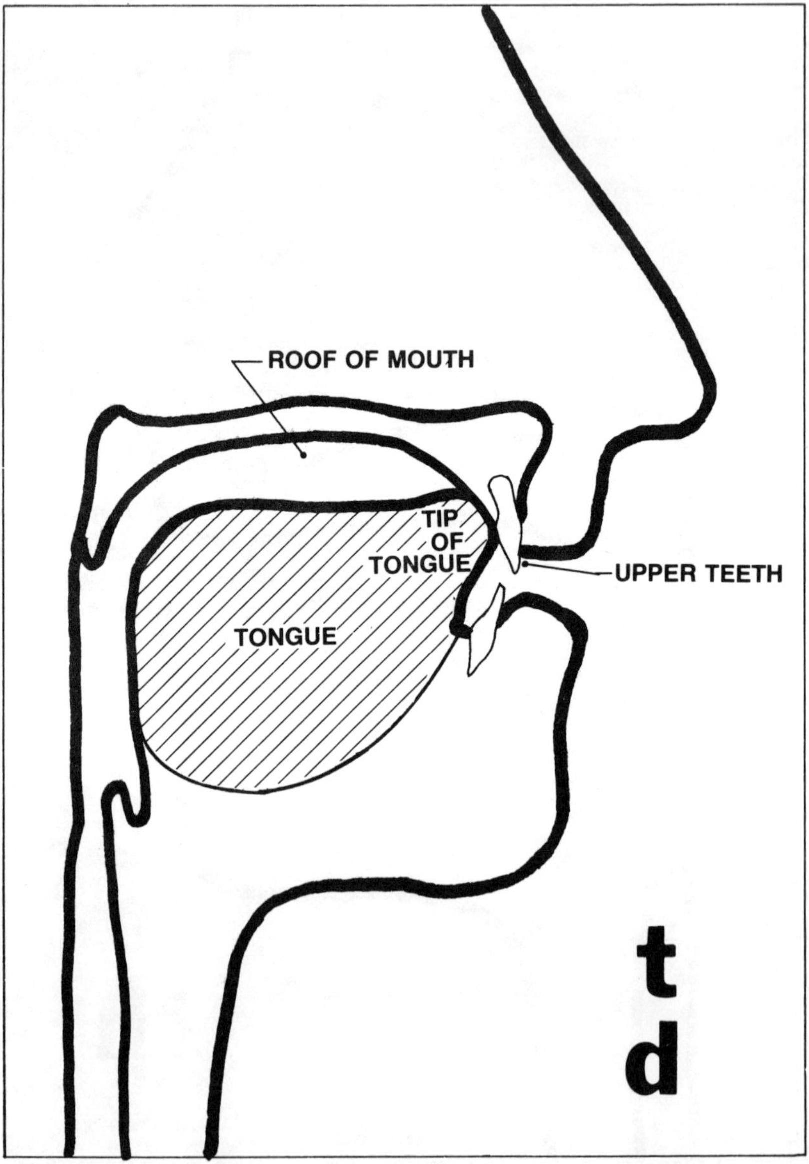

Figure 11.8. *t*, *d:* Tip of tongue is pressed against upper gums just behind teeth, then released sharply; *t* is voiceless; *d* is voiced.

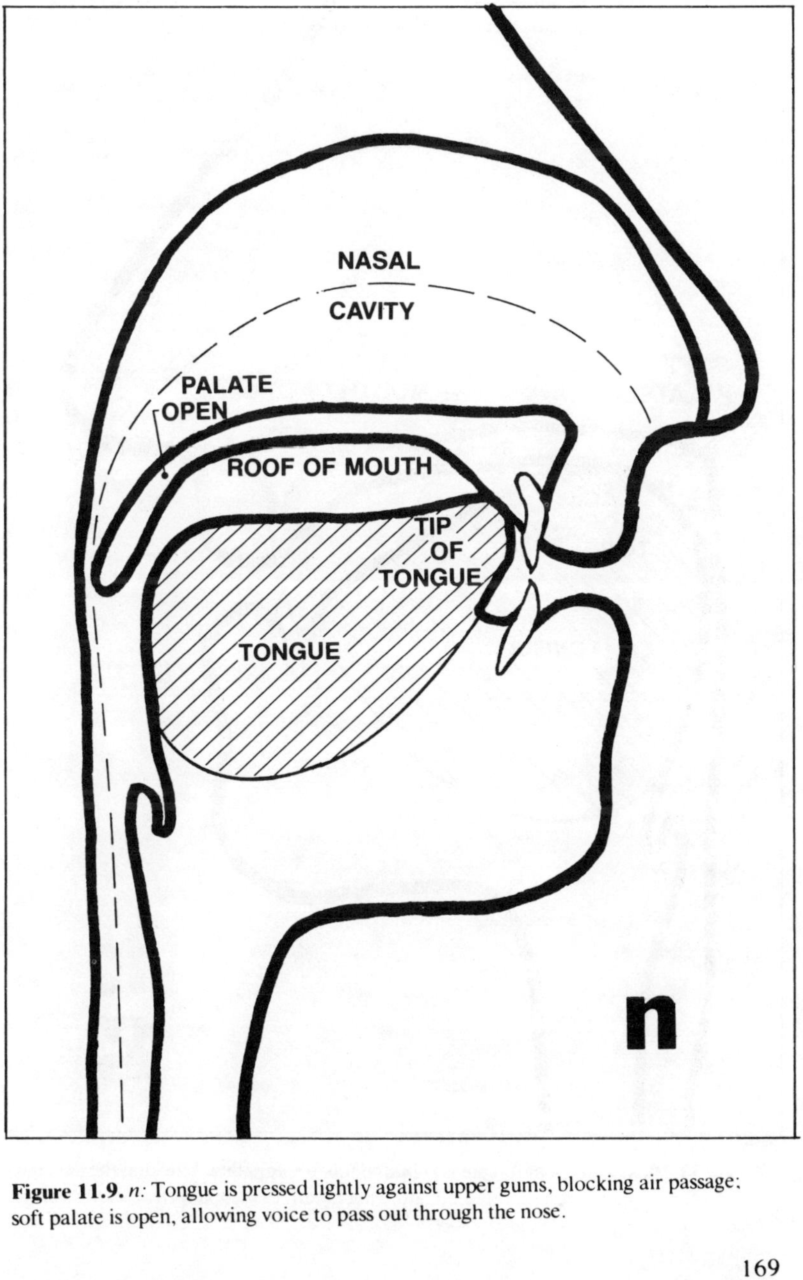

Figure 11.9. *n:* Tongue is pressed lightly against upper gums, blocking air passage; soft palate is open, allowing voice to pass out through the nose.

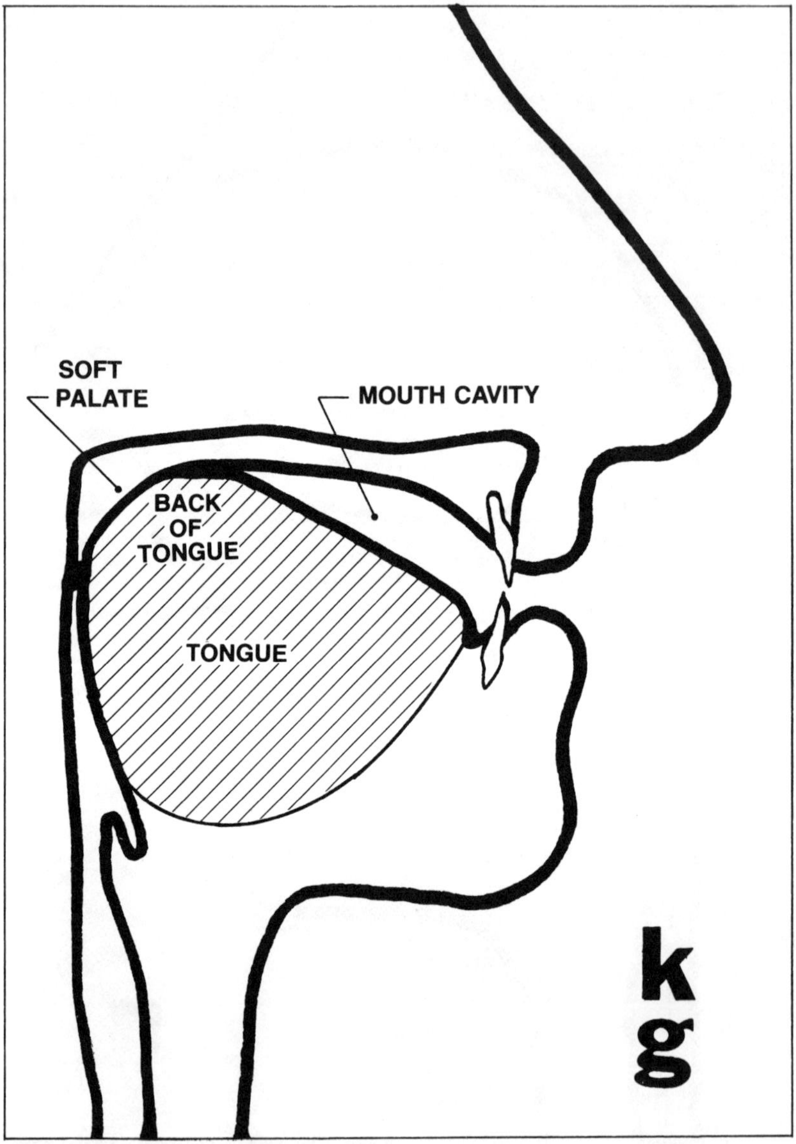

Figure 11.10. *k, g:* Back of tongue is raised to touch soft palate, blocking the passage of air; then back of tongue is released, allowing breath to escape with an explosive sound; *k* is voiceless; *g* is voiced.

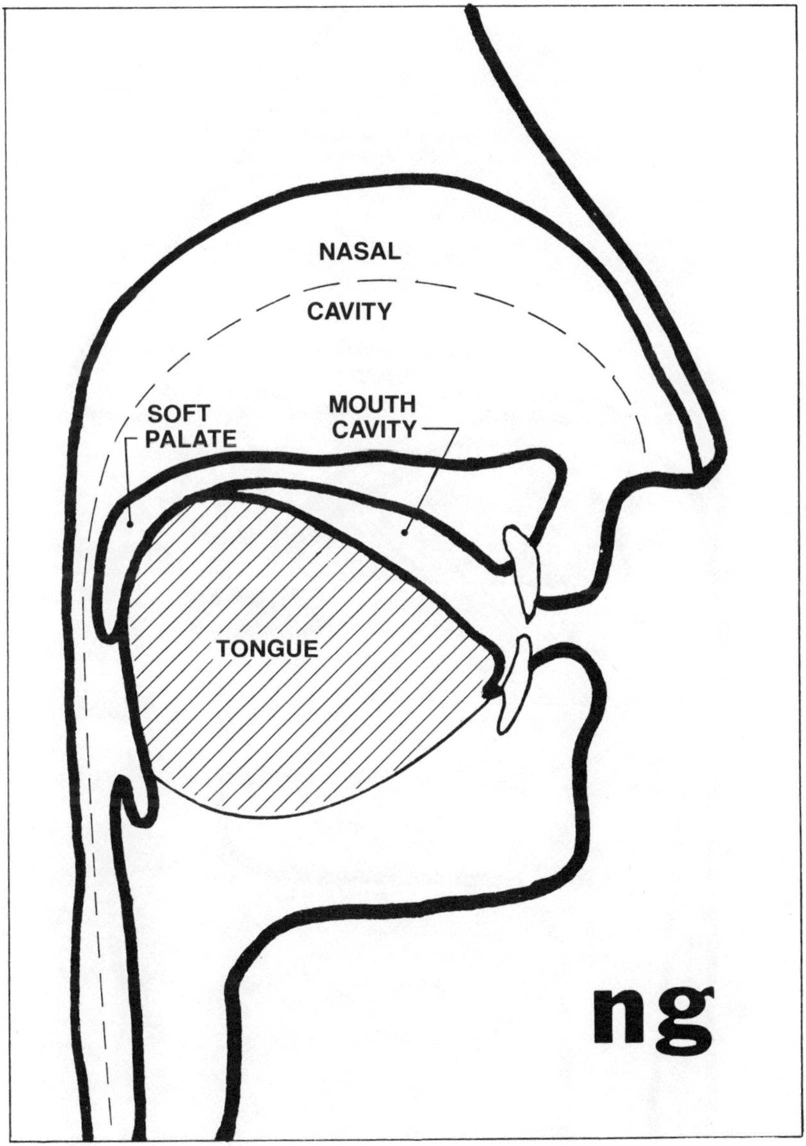

Figure 11.11. *ng:* Back of tongue is pressed against soft palate; soft palate is open to allow voiced air to pass out through the nose.

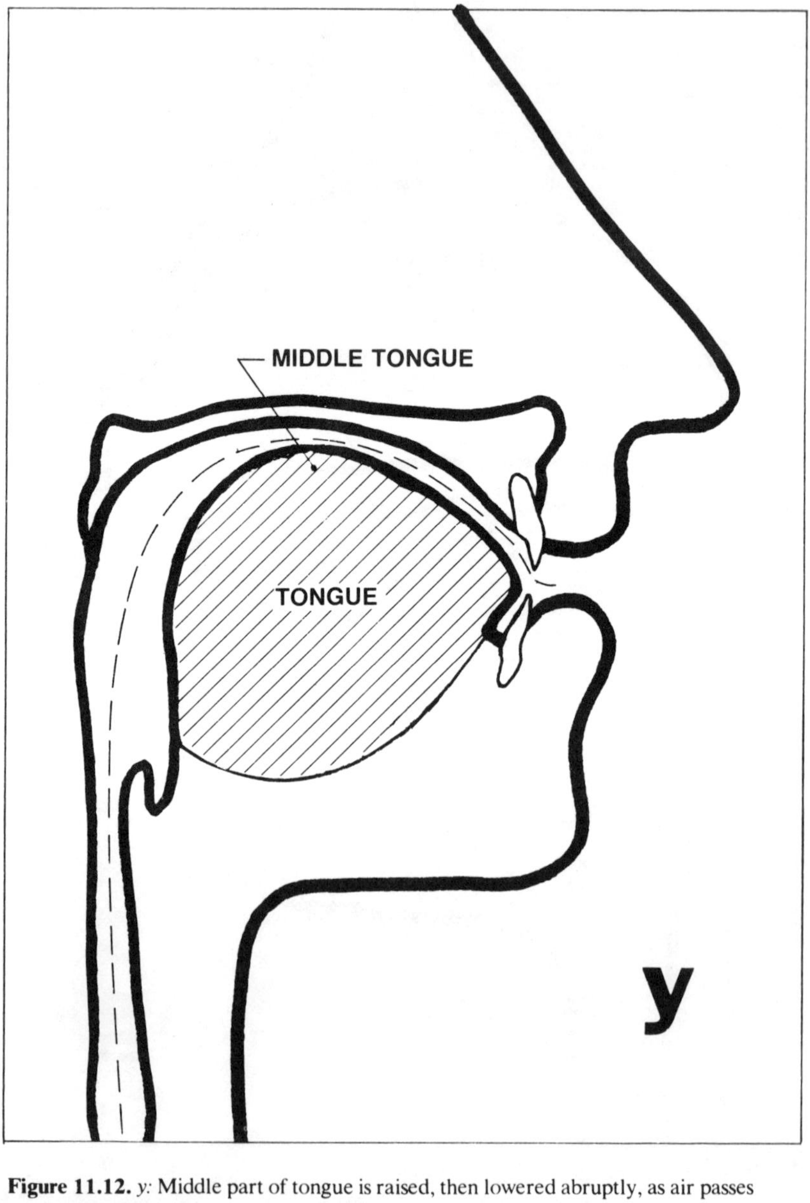

Figure 11.12. *y:* Middle part of tongue is raised, then lowered abruptly, as air passes out through the mouth.

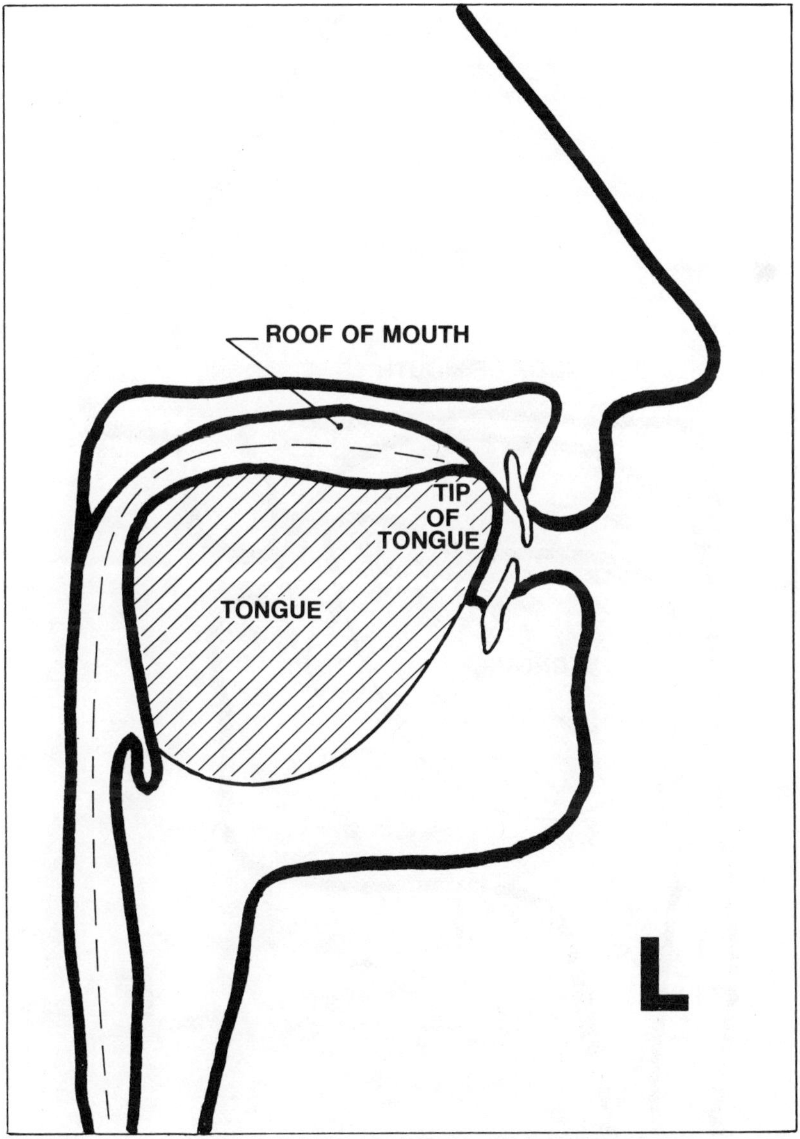

Figure 11.13. *l:* Tip of tongue is pressed against upper teeth ridge; air passes out through opening between sides of tongue and side teeth.

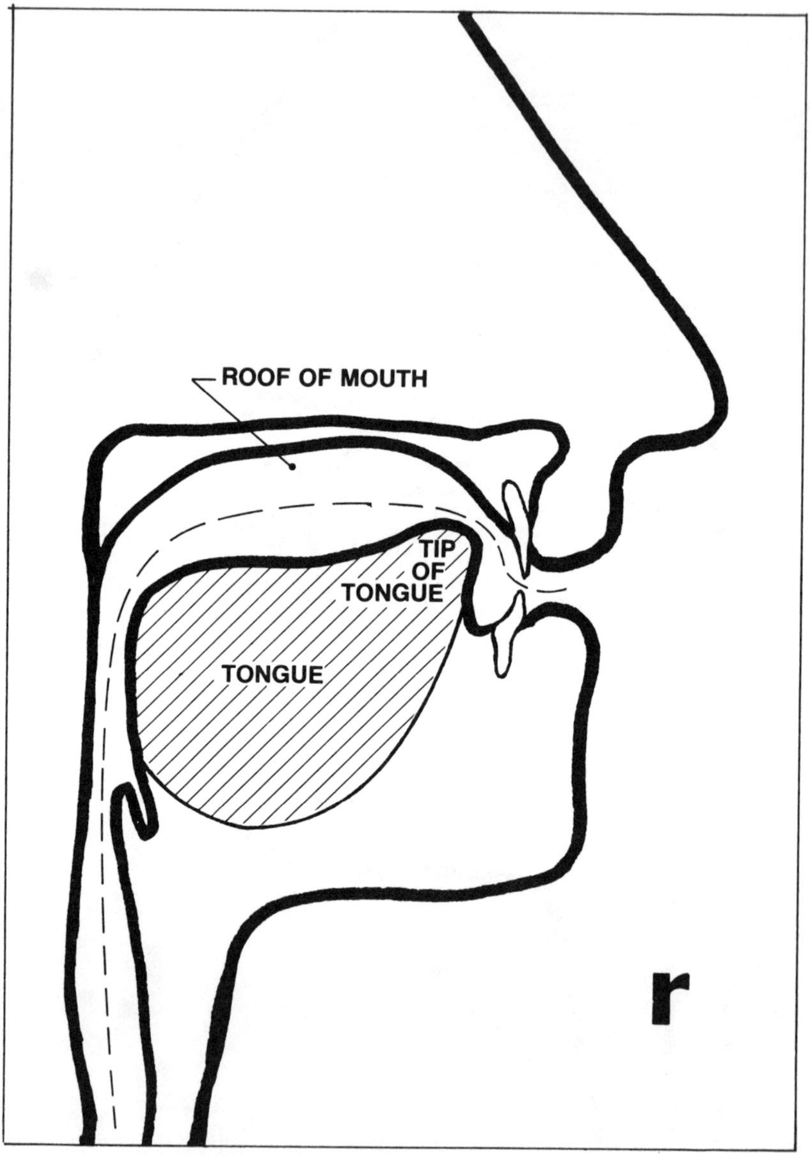

Figure 11.14. *r:* Tip of tongue is raised and turned slightly backward; sides of tongue touch upper side teeth, causing air to flow out over tip of tongue.

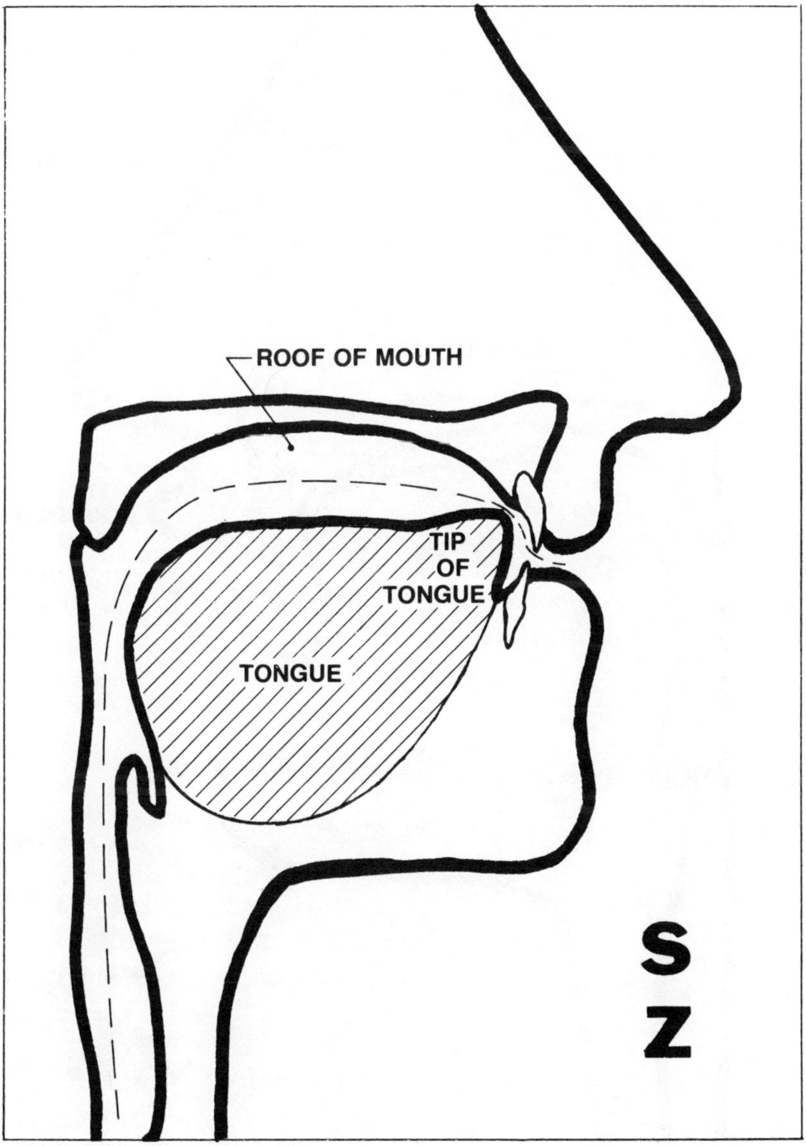

Figure 11.15. *s, z:* Tongue, wide and thin, touches roof of mouth at sides; tongue tip is raised, with a very narrow groove in center, through which the air passes out of the mouth; *s* is voiceless; *z* is voiced.

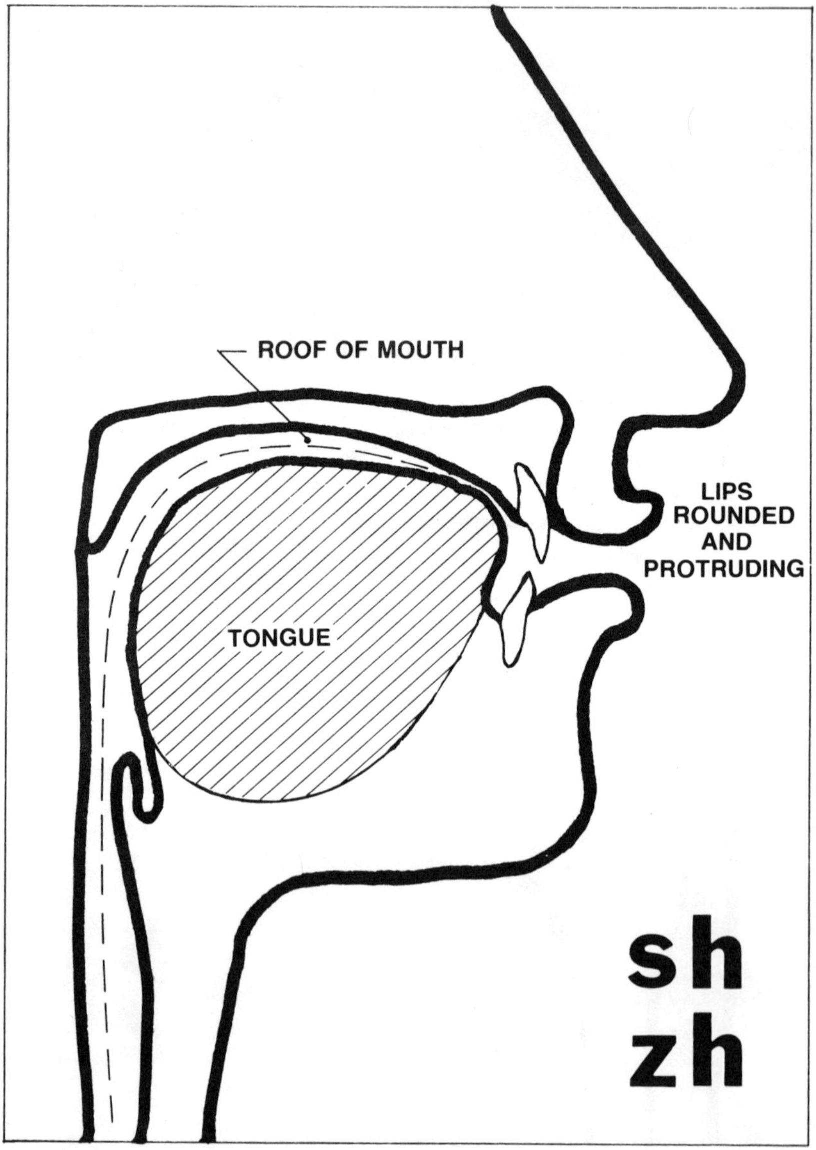

Figure 11.16. *sh, zh:* Tongue is positioned as for *s* and *z,* except that tip is drawn back a little farther; lips are rounded and protruding; *sh* is voiceless; *zh* (as in trea*s*ure) is voiced.

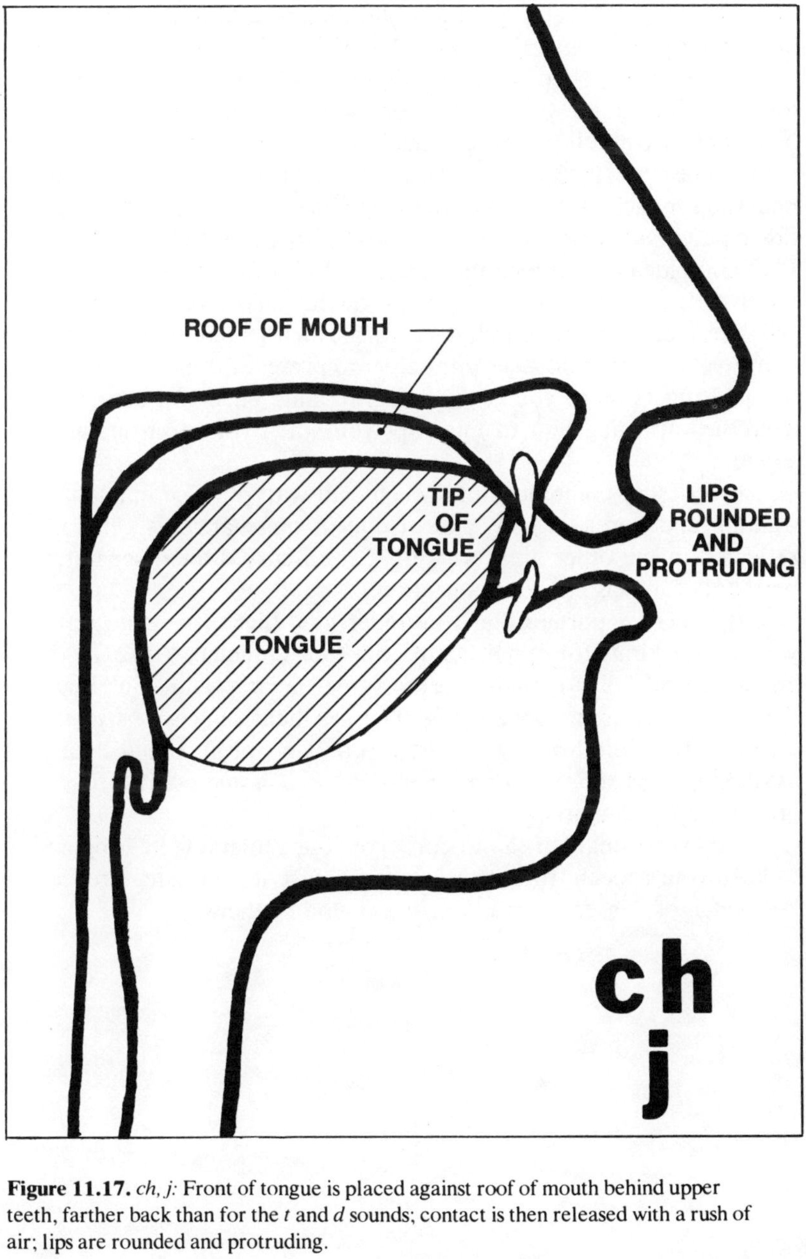

Figure 11.17. *ch, j:* Front of tongue is placed against roof of mouth behind upper teeth, farther back than for the *t* and *d* sounds; contact is then released with a rush of air; lips are rounded and protruding.

stream of air passing through the small opening between your tongue tip and your front teeth. For the *s* and *z* sounds, it may help you to begin with your tongue tip placed flat against the ridge behind your upper front teeth. Then place a toothpick on top of the center of your tongue tip, making a very small opening for the air to pass through. Your helper can tell you when your *s* and *z* sounds are correct. For your home speech training periods, use a drill book that contains material for each of the sounds of the language. An excellent book of this type is *Fundamentals of Voice and Diction,* by Lyle V. Mayer. It's a good idea to start with the sound by itself first. Then, when your family helper tells you that you are producing it correctly, proceed to syllables including the sound, then words, then sentences, and finally conversational speech. Ask your helper to present the material to you by speaking close to your ear or hearing aid. Then you repeat the exercises, allowing him to interrupt you when you misarticulate a sound.

It is best to combine your speech drill with practice in auditory training and lipreading. A gain in one of these areas is generally reflected in the other areas as well. I've discussed them separately here only for reasons of organization.

It is very important that you understand that there is no do-it-yourself substitute for a well-qualified speech clinician. You *need* the guidance and help of such a professional person, and you should make every effort to obtain this. The self-help suggestions in this chapter are offered *only* as a last resort if no professional help is available, or as *supplementary* material for at-home practice if you are receiving regular speech therapy.

Do everything you can to conserve your remaining hearing and to keep your speech from deteriorating before it's too late. I repeat: An ounce of conservation is worth a pound of therapy.

12

How can I cope with the social and emotional problems I face?

Once there was a young girl who had very crooked teeth. It didn't really bother her much at first, but whenever she looked in the mirror, she was vaguely dissatisfied with what she saw. She couldn't admit to herself that she didn't like the way she looked, so she started keeping her mouth closed when she looked in the mirror. One day, she heard the boy next door say, "Here comes old horse-teeth." After that, she tried to avoid smiling whenever she was around people. It wasn't long before her friends began to shut her out of their circle. She thought it was because her teeth made her ugly, never guessing that the real reason had to do with her defensive attitude and her refusal to smile. Whenever she heard people whispering or talking in small groups, she was sure they were talking about her and her ugly teeth. Pretty soon, she started avoiding social situations because it was such a strain to be constantly hiding her teeth. Her parents suggested braces, but she was afraid that would just call attention to her "handicap." She became depressed, and that scared her because she couldn't understand *why* she wasn't happy. Soon she began to think of herself as a mouth full of ugly teeth instead of a normal girl with a problem, and she became more and more depressed and more and more withdrawn.

This little anecdote illustrates some of the social and emotional problems hard-of-hearing and deaf people face. Let me say at the outset that there's no typical hard-of-hearing personality. Each person reacts in his own unique way to his hearing problem. And let me assure you that I'm not going to minimize or belittle your feelings. They are very real and also very *natural* reactions to a difficult coping situation. Your hearing problem is likely to make you feel depressed, and for good reason. It may exaggerate any natural tendencies you have toward extroversion or introversion. Your suspicions that other people are talking about you are a perfectly natural reaction. People with normal hearing often feel that way when they can't hear the conversations of people around them, too. And, since we all tend to avoid painful situations, it's normal to withdraw from social contacts that cause strain and frustration. There's one more reason why I'm not going to belittle your social and emotional problems. That is the fact that people who hear normally really *can* be cruel and prejudiced against the hard of hearing. Many of them really *don't* understand your problems and really *are* indifferent to the plight of the hard-of-hearing adult. I wish it were not that way, but I'd be deceiving you if I tried to deny it.

Well, then, is there anything I can do to ease the unhappiness and frustration I feel? Yes. Right now, you may feel that you're locked in a jail—one that is caused partly by your hearing loss with its resulting problems of communication, partly by your own ailing self-image, and partly by the misunderstanding of other people. In order to get out, you're going to need three things: (1) a key, which is total *acceptance* of your hearing loss; (2) a sliding door, which is a thorough *understanding* of *why* you feel the way you do; (3) and some legwork, which involves some practical, down-to-earth kinds of positive *action* you can take toward freeing yourself from the sound-barrier jail. In this chapter, we'll consider all three of these tools. You may well find this to be the most personally valuable chapter in the whole book!

Why do you consider total acceptance of my hearing problem the key to breaking the sound barrier? Because, as long as you refuse to admit to yourself that your hearing defect is real, as long as you hold out unrealistic hope for a miraculous cure, as long as you try to bluff your way through social situations, hoping to hide your loss, you are adding unnecessary strain to the already difficult stresses your loss imposes. The "canker sore" of nonacceptance will fester and grow below the surface of your consciousness, increasing your unhappiness and poisoning your self-image. No one can help you solve a problem you refuse to admit.

So your first step, and the one on which all progress depends, is to admit to yourself that you do not hear well. You probably would not be reading this book if you had not already taken that step. But are you still clinging to hope for a cure, or at least for improvement in the physical part of your hearing ability? If your hearing specialist is convinced that your loss is permanent, consult another otologist if you wish. If they both agree that there is nothing more that can be done to improve your hearing, then accept that verdict as final, irreversible. Only then can you begin to develop a positive attitude of coping realistically with a very real problem.

Next, learn as much as you can about hearing loss in general and your own loss in particular. The extreme significance of this factor is the motivating force behind this book.

Especially if your loss is mild, you may be tempted to try to ignore it. You may consider it to be a disagreeable sign of weakness or aging, and so feel a strong need to keep others from finding out about it. But you pay a high emotional price for such false pride. Joseph Sataloff describes the results:

> Such a person, to keep up with a conversation, makes strenuous listening efforts and fills in hearing gaps by guessing, while he carefully conceals his frustration by acting particularly pleasant and affable. His efforts to "save face" lead to numerous embarrassing situations, become fatiguing and lead to nervousness, irritability and instability.[1]

But it doesn't have to be this way. D. A. Ramsdell sounds this positive note:

> The first step toward surmounting the difficulty is to admit it frankly and realistically. Much of the tension of social situations is eased for the deafened as well as for others if the impairment is regarded as factually and objectively as the need for glasses. Society accepts glasses for impaired vision and will accept with equal readiness the wearing of a hearing aid and also the need for face-to-face conversation to facilitate lipreading . . . by those whose impairment is too severe for a hearing aid.[2]

So, when you meet someone new, *tell him,* right away, that you have a hearing loss, and ask him to speak slowly but not to shout, and to look at you as he talks so you can read his lips. This may be hard the first few times, but force yourself to do it. This way, he'll know that your problem is hearing and not snobbishness or retardation, and he'll be relieved to know how best to communicate with you. If you've noticed that people seem to avoid you at social gatherings, you'll find this happening less often once you take this approach. It also relieves you of the burden of trying to bluff, which doesn't work anyway! Here are the words of a severely deafened otologist, who *knows* how you feel because he's been there:

> I wasted from five to ten of what should have been the best years of my life as a selfish, depressed and self-pitying man. . . . I was like an ostrich with my head in the sand trying to conceal something which everyone already knew. It was not until I finally accepted my deafness as an unalterable fact and acquired the determination to overcome my handicap, that I really began to enjoy life again. . . .[3]

There's one more thing we need to talk about regarding acceptance of your problem. Let's be completely realistic about this. Some people are still going to be inconsiderate, no matter what you do. It may help you to know that many such people have low self-esteem—they have to step on other people to build up their own egos. Or they may be simply unthinking and hurt you unintentionally because they don't understand your problem. This, too, you must accept and even expect. Sure, it hurts, but knowing what causes it may help you to rise above the pettiness and lack of understanding. Being able to do this will help you to grow a little as a human being. Sataloff says, "Although this indifference is cruel, it does require the hard-of-hearing person to develop a usefully independent and objective attitude toward his handicap."[4]

But I've accepted my loss as final and admitted it freely to others, and I still feel depressed, sometimes suspicious, and lonely. Why? These emotional states are very common and natural tagalongs that come with hearing loss. Fortunately, just being able to understand *why* you feel as you do can take you a long way toward shaking off the hurt you feel. Often, people who have hearing handicaps blame themselves for not being able to "snap out of it." They think that, if they were only brave enough, they'd be able to control their feelings. Guilt feelings of this kind are not only unjustified, but they can be downright destructive. There are some very logical and subtle *reasons* for the way you feel, and these have nothing to do with weakness or lack of willpower. We'll get into those reasons in a minute, but first, we need to differentiate between the feelings of those who were born deaf and those who acquired thier hearing losses in later life.

Who has more emotional problems—the congenitally deaf or those who lost their hearing later? The psychological problems of the two groups are different. Both have communication troubles, which naturally give rise to feelings of isolation, but those whose deafness occurred before they acquired language skills obviously have a bigger problem in this area. As we've said before, language is learned in an unconscious way, through the sense of hearing. Deprived of that, some deaf people never learn to effectively communicate with hearing people. This sets them apart. On the other hand, they may have an advantage over those with *acquired* losses, in that they never have to adjust to the shock of losing something they once had, of having their world "shrink."

How does severity of loss affect emotional adjustment? The greater the loss, the more serious the communication problem is. Surprisingly, though, some people with mild losses suffer more than those whose impairments are profound. Why? Because they are more likely to deny their handicap, to bluff their way through conversations, and to refuse a hearing aid for fear of calling attention to their problem. All of these defenses place heavy, unnecessary strain on the individual. They make him nervous and irritable and cause extreme fatigue. When you're fighting something and trying to hide it, when you're worn out from strain, you're more vulnerable to frustration and depression.

What causes my feeling of depression? The underlying cause may be something of which you are completely unaware. Ramsdell describes three psychological levels of hearing: the primitive level, the warning level, and the social level.[5] The greatest cause of your depression may lie on the primitive level.

What is this primitive level of hearing? It's all of the background noises that we respond to unconciously even though we don't realize we hear them—the furnace going on and off, a clock ticking, people moving around in other rooms, our own footsteps, cars going by outside, etc.

Why are these sounds so important? As Ramsdell says, "these incidental noises maintain our feeling of being part of a living world and contribute to our own sense of being alive. We are not conscious of the important role which these background sounds play in our comfortable merging of ourselves with the life around us, because we are not aware of them. Nor is the deaf man aware that he has lost these sounds; he only knows that *he feels as if the world were dead*. . . . The loss of this feeling of relationship with the world is the major cause of the well-recognized feeling of 'deadness' and also of the depression that permeates the suddenly deafened and, to a lesser degree, those in whom deafness develops gradually."[6]

So what can I do about it? I'm going to quote Ramsdell again because he says it better than I could:

> *An extremely important step toward relieving the characteristic depression is taken when the deaf person realizes the reason for his emotional state.* The realization it-

> self makes his depression more objective and thereby makes it possible for him to cope with it without bewilderment or self-blame. As long as he is blind to its causes, he suffers from the same vague feelings of discomfort that characterize the early stages of a disease before the symptoms have yet developed clearly. Diagnosis does not instantly remove a disease, but it makes the proper treatment possible. Similarly, knowing the cause of depression does not remove it, but fortunately *the mere understanding of the reason for a feeling state does much psychologically to relieve its intensity.*

Because this primitive level of hearing is so essential to your feeling of well-being, it's reason enough to wear your hearing aid, even if your loss is so severe that the device doesn't make it possible for you to understand speech. I'll give you some practical suggestions later in the chapter that may help you to compensate for your "deadened world."

What is the second psychological level of hearing? Ramsdell calls it the 'warning level.' On the *primitive* level, we react to background noises *unconsciously,* but there are also many sounds that we *notice consciously* and that cause us to take some appropriate action. The child who hears his mother coming up the stairs may shove his cutting-and-pasting mess under the bed. (In our house, it's more likely to be a pet frog or mud turtle in a shoe-box cage!) We go to the door when we hear a knock or answer the phone when it rings. We get out of bed (sometimes!) when we hear the alarm ring, step out of the street when a car honks, go to the basement if the tornado siren blows. Hearing also tells us what *direction* sounds are coming from. If you have a severe hearing loss in only one ear, you will have trouble determining the direction from which sounds are coming. When we can't hear sounds that keep us informed about what's going on around us, we may feel somewhat insecure. Still, the problems caused by inability to hear at this *warning* level are less severe than those caused by loss of primitive-level hearing. Flashing lights may be substituted for doorbells and telephone bells. (See Chapter 15.) Becoming *visually* aware can partially make up for loss of directional hearing. Except for some vague feelings of insecurity, loss at this second level of hearing is not likely to be the cause of your greatest emotional problems.

What is the third psychological level of hearing? This is the social or symbolic level, which involves the use of the spoken word for communication. Almost every person who has a hearing loss has some trouble on this level. If your hearing loss occurred before the age of two, you know the struggle of trying to learn language without hearing. The chances are, if your loss is severe and lifelong, you have come to depend heavily on manual communication (sign language and fingerspelling). Early use of manual communication is effective in helping the child form language concepts, but it does make it difficult for him to interact with the hearing world. Yet the goal of oral language for *all* deaf people is unrealistic. You may need an interpreter to help you communicate with hearing people who don't know sign language. You will naturally feel isolated at times. Later in the chapter, I'll offer some down-to-earth suggestions for coping with these feelings.

If your hearing loss developed later in life, your communication problems may be particularly distressing to you. You miss the easy give-and-take and emotional release of chatting comfortably with a friend. You may be ill at ease in group situations because it's just too frustrating to try to keep up with the rapidly moving conversations. You may begin to avoid social activities and withdraw into yourself. All of these reactions (which are very *normal*) tend to increase your feelings of depression and loneliness. You may even become overly suspicious of your family and friends.

What makes me so suspicious? All of us have a tendency, when we notice people talking but can't tell what they're saying, to wonder if they're talking about us. If we're especially sensitive about some fault we have (like the girl with the crooked teeth), we begin to *expect* people to be critical of us. When we hear laughter, we think we're being ridiculed. When we notice a frown or a sour look, we assume it is directed at us. This is even more likely to happen if we're already feeling depressed. So you can see why, if you're a sensitive person, your hearing loss may easily bring out these feelings of suspicion. Just knowing *why* you feel this way may help you to feel less guilty about your suspicious feelings.

Then, too, if you can develop more interests that are centered outside of yourself, you will be less concerned with what other people are saying. Then you can be more objective about the whole thing. The suggestions that follow will help you, if you're willing to give them a try.

Now that I understand why I feel the way I do, can you give me some practical suggestions for overcoming my painful emotions? Yes. An article in *Psychology Today* magazine describes depression as "a fall into helplessness."[8] The author explains that we become depressed when we feel, for one reason or another, that we are no longer in full control of our lives. Loss of hearing can certainly make you feel that way! The best antidote for this state of mind, then, is to *take some kind of positive action.* It doesn't really matter too much *what* that action is, as long as it gives us the feeling that we're actually *doing* something about our problems. Action (any positive kind) can replace that falling sensation with a climbing sensation that will help to dispel the darkness. In previous chapters, we've already talked about some kinds of action you can take (getting a hearing aid, learning to lipread, practicing auditory training, getting vocational counseling, etc.). Here are some other actions you can take that are more specifically directed toward your social and emotional problems.

1. If your depression is severe, or your feelings of loneliness and suspicion are acute, or your hearing impairment is creating problems within your family, by all means arrange for psychological counseling. Ask your otologist, audiologist, or speech and hearing clinician to recommend a counselor who is familiar with the problems of the hard of hearing. If possible, get the whole family involved in this. They're sure to benefit from a better understanding of your feelings, and they, too, may be having difficulty handling some of their own reactions to your hearing impairment.

2. Next, I'd suggest that you set some new and absorbing goals for yourself and then get busy on achieving them. They may be related to your hearing loss (e.g., improving your lipreading skills) or they may not. A few years ago, I wrote an article about this very thing for *Guideposts* magazine. I've received the editors' permission to reproduce it here for you. It has been reprinted many times, and I've received numerous letters from people who have said it has helped them to get out of an emotional slump. I hope it will help you, too.

How To Aim Yourself

It was my thirty-fifth birthday and all day I had been struggling against the gnawing awareness that my life was half over. What did I have to show for a life half-spent? I realized that what I really needed more than anything else was a feeling of achievement. I guess we all need that—almost as much as we need food and water.

As I cleared the table, I thought of how often I had heard myself say, "Gee, I really intended to do that," or "I'd do it if I just had more time," but I never seemed to *get* anywhere. Maybe my aim was wrong.

That one word, *aim,* hovered strangely in my thoughts for a minute before it connected unexpectedly with the memory of my first bowling lesson, given me by my father. Strange that something as unprofound as a bowling technique could rescue me from the quicksand of unproductivity, but as soon as I started applying a bowling formula to my life goals, things began to happen. I earned my master's degree, gained a pilot's license and launched a career in writing, in addition to reaching some other less ambitious goals. But more important, it helped me exchange my vague feeling of unworthiness for the bold hope that maybe my life could really count for something after all.

I'd like to share the ways in which the "aim yourself" technique has worked for me, in the hope that it might help you, too.

The first step in my father's bowling formula is: Pick a spot just in front of you that's in line with the center pin. When I applied that advice to my life, I realized I had to aim toward one goal at a time and that each goal had to be exact. My vague desire to be a better housekeeper was not good enough, I had to really pin it down and resolve to "clean out the linen closet and the coat closet *today.*"

I also learned to choose goals that I could start on right now and accomplish within a limited time. I had always thought that someday I'd like to go back to college and get a master's degree, but the prospect was so overwhelming that I kept putting it off. So instead of aiming for my degree, I signed up for just one class. Aiming for a spot "just in front of me" made it easier to begin. We need long-term goals, too, but I have found that we reach broader, distant goals by the route of today's well-aimed single steps.

Since the "spot" must be "in line with the center pin," I try to test each goal with these questions: Will it make me more nearly the kind of person I want to be? Will its accomplishment further my long-term goals? Is it significant enough to spend part of myself on?

After I have selected a goal that is exact, short-term, and in line with my "center pin" goals, I'm ready for step two: Aim your whole self toward the goal. In bowling, golf, archery, or any other sport where aim is important, the whole body has to "follow through." Single-mindedness is just as important in aiming for short-term goals in life. Here are some tricks that have helped me keep my attention focused on my current goals. As soon as I set a goal for myself, I do something *right then* toward its accomplishment. When I resolved to redecorate the bedroom, I bought some green paint. When I decided to take flying lessons, I made an appointment for my first lesson.

Next, I tell someone about my goal. This makes it harder for me to talk myself out of it later. Then I make three copies of the goal, including time limit, placing these reminders by things I use every day—in my silverware drawer, on the refrigerator door, in the coat pocket that holds my keys. Every time I run across one of these reminders during the day, I try to stop what I'm doing and make some further effort toward my goal. If I can't stop, I can at least plan what my next step will be and exactly when I will do it.

After I have done everything I can toward the accomplishment of a particular goal, I take the third and final step: Let go of the ball. I turn the outcome over to God, knowing that, just as there are physical laws that make a bowling ball keep rolling once it's started, there are also spiritual laws that take over for us after we have chosen an exact goal and aimed our whole self toward it. Sometimes it's hard for me to let go and let God, but I have learned that if I can do just that, the ball I started rolling will continue on its way with the help of God and by His sure laws.

I still give up on goals sometimes. My housekeeping never did improve all that much, and my thumb is not getting any greener; but I find that I'm succeeding far more often than I used to, because the formula keeps my aim short, direct and concentrated. And it's the very best remedy in the world for that I-never-seem-to-get-anywhere feeling. Goal bowling, anyone?[9]

3. In addition to professional counseling and "goal bowling," you may need to do some homework on your own self-concept. Remember the girl with the crooked teeth who began to think of herself as "a mouthful of ugly teeth, instead of as a normal girl with a problem"? People with impaired hearing often develop a similar lopsided view of themselves. Remind yourself that *you are not your hearing loss!* You are far more normal than abnormal. But my telling you that will not change the way you view yourself unless you're willing to spend some time working on your thoughts. Abe Lincoln was right. Most people *are* about as happy as they make up their minds to be. If you'll think about it, you'll realize that it's not what *happens* to us that makes us happy people or unhappy people. It's how we *react* to what happens to us. And we *can* consciously *decide* how we're going to react to a given situation. Most of us bob up and down through our disappointments and frustrations, clinging to the sides of leaky boats. But it doesn't have to be that way. We can use our thoughts as bailing buckets to keep our boats from sinking.

That sounds good, but how does it work? Try this. First, make out a list of all the things you can think of that you do well. Then write down, on another list, things that give you pleasure that don't require you to use your sense of hearing. Now set aside fifteen or twenty minutes a day for thought conditioning. (This is so important that you could even borrow time from your daily speech-lipreading-auditory training period on very busy days.) Go into a room by yourself, and get into a comfortable, relaxed, sitting position. (Don't lie down. You might fall asleep!) Now, close your eyes and start to think about *one* thing from the lists you've made. Picture yourself actually doing that one thing. Make your mental picture as vivid and real as possible.

For instance, if you like to fish, picture yourself sitting by the lake, line in the water. "Listen" to the soft breeze rustling the leaves of the trees. (Are they elms? Cottonwoods? Birches?) "See" the soft ripples on the water; "smell" the scent of wild plum blossoms in the air; "feel" the tug of a fish on your line. Reel him in and *savor* the feeling of accomplishment and satisfaction your catch brings. Mentally congratulate yourself on your success. See yourself as a person who can and does perform—who knows how to achieve and follows through on that ability. If negative thoughts creep in, gently bail them out, filling the hole with the pleasant scene you're experiencing. Continue in this way for fifteen or twenty minutes and then stop. (You don't want to *live* in a fantasy world—just "visit" it once or twice a day.) The next time you do this, choose a different item from your lists. If you'll set aside a definite time for this every day, you'll soon find that the positive feelings you generate will begin to carry over into your everyday life.

4. If you have a hearing aid, by all means wear it as much as possible. If you're having trouble adjusting to it, reread the suggestions in Chapter 8. Even if the aid doesn't make your hearing adequate for easy communication, the background sounds it brings in will help at that primitive level of hearing to give your world a feeling of aliveness. Your hearing aid is valuable to you when you're out in public, not only because it amplifies sound, but also because, if it's visible, it serves as a sign and a reminder to others that your problem is physical and not intellectual. This will relieve you of some of your feelings of insecurity.

5. To avoid brooding and self-pity, try to fill your leisure time with some creative activity or hobby. You may want to take up ceramics or needlepoint, stamp collecting or rock polishing and jewelry making, to mention only a few of the possibilities. My husband, who is hard of hearing, bought an old Model A and spends much of his free time restoring and improving it. (Our garage looks like a junk yard, but Rex's outlook on life is in pretty good shape. I'll trade a spic-and-span garage for a happy husband any day!)

6. Read some good books by and/or about hard-of-hearing and deaf people who have learned to cope with their handicaps. It will do you a mountain of good to realize that others have struggled with the same problems you have. If they can overcome, so can you. Some examples are:

I'm Deaf Too: 12 Deaf Americans, edited by Frank Bowe and Martin Sternberg, published by National Association of the Deaf, 814 Thayer Avenue, Silver Spring, MD 20910.

A Deaf Adult Speaks Out, by Leo M. Jacobs, published by Gallaudet College Press, Washington, DC 20002.

Hearing is Believing, by Marie Hays Heiner, published by World Publishing Company, Cleveland, Ohio.

Cotton in My Ears, by Frances Warfield, published by Viking, New York, New York.

Let's Hear It! by George W. Frankel, published by Stratford House, New York, New York.

7. Join a local organization for the hearing impaired, or, if there isn't one in your community, start one. Even if your community is small, there are probably at least a few others who share your problem. Put an ad in the paper.

8. National organizations can also give you a feeling of belonging, and many of them publish magazines that have articles about the problems you share with other subscribers. See Chapter 14 for a listing of these organizations.

9. Here are some tips that can help you in social situations. I've mentioned some of them before, but they are worth repeating.

a. Tell new acquaintances about your loss immediately. Don't be afraid to ask them to face you when speaking and to speak in a normal tone of voice, without exaggerating their lip movements. *But—*

b. Don't imply that it's their fault that you can't hear them.

c. Develop your sense of humor. Don Pettingill, who has been deaf since childhood, says this: "Some of the finest senses of humor I have ever enjoyed are possessed by deaf persons, even those who can't speak a word or lip-read any better. By golly, we have to have a good laugh once in a while or we fast become cynics or worse."[10]

d. If your communication problem is severe, you may need an interpreter for certain occasions. If you don't have anyone who can help you in this way, write to Registry of Interpreters of the Deaf. The address is given in Chapter 14.

e. If you have a career problem, Chapter 13 will give you some helpful suggestions for coping with this.

f. There's another kind of action you can take that will not only help your morale, but may also bring about added benefits to the deaf population. I'm talking about political action. Frederick Schreiber of the National As-

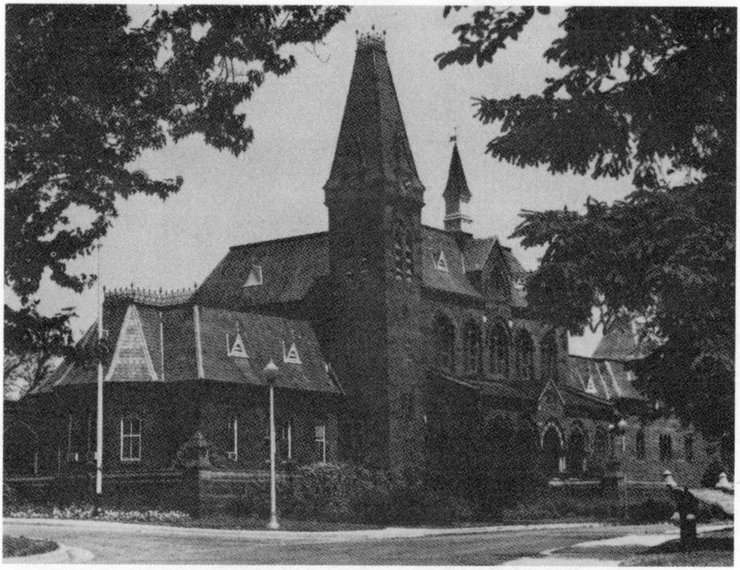

Figure 12.1. Chapel Hall at Gallaudet College was built in 1871 and has been designated a National Historic Landmark by the National Park Service. (Gallaudet College photo.)

sociation of the Deaf spells out the need: "If the deaf are to get the kind of service they need and the protection they are entitled to under the laws of our country, they will have to become much more involved in politics than has been the case heretofore."[11]

If you're interested, I'd suggest that you write to Mr. Schreiber, c/o National Association of the Deaf (address given in Chapter 14.) Ask him what you can do to help.

10. In addition to the above suggestions, I would urge you to try to strengthen and deepen your religious faith. In my own life, I've found that there is no better remedy for feelings of depression and isolation than prayer and meditation. Knowing that God will never forsake me has carried me through many stormy seas in my life. If you have drifted away from your own religious faith over the years, you may

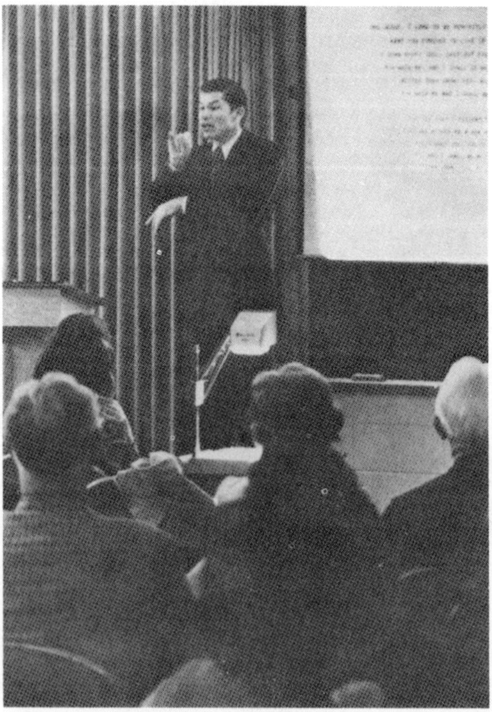

Figure 12.2. The Reverend Duane King, conducting services using sign language and visual materials, at Christ's Church of the Deaf in Council Bluffs, Iowa.

find that steering your life back to sacred waters may help to keep your "leaky boat" on top of the water.

At least fifteen different religious denominations now have special ministries for the deaf and hard of hearing. Your community may have a church whose services feature visual aids (such as sign language, projected slides, printed signs, etc.) to help the hearing handicapped.

Deaf Missions of Council Bluffs, Iowa, offers a gold mine of religious materials for use by hearing-impaired people and those who work with them. (See address in Chapter 14.)

Books can also be an excellent source of inspiration. Here are a few that have been especially helpful to me in my spiritual and psychological quest for meaning:

Beyond Our Selves, by Catherine Marshall, published by McGraw Hill, New York.

Breakthrough to Life, by Hans Hofmann, published by Beacon Press, Boston.

Coming into Existence, by Raymond Rogers, published by Dell Publishing Co., New York.

Hotline to Heaven, by Frances Gardner Hunter, published by Warner Press, Anderson, Indiana.

The Miracle of Mind Power, by Dan Custer, published by Prentice-Hall, Englewood Cliffs, New Jersey.

Psycho-cybernetics, by Maxwell Maltz, published by Prentice-Hall, Inc., Englewood Cliffs, New Jersey.

The Struggle of the Soul, by Lewis Joseph Sherrill, published by the Macmillan Company, New York.

The Taste of New Wine, by Keith Miller, published by Word Books, Waco, Texas.

Thoreau's *Walden* and the poetry of William Blake and Gerard Manley Hopkins also provide me with special inspiration.

You can probably find most of these, as well as others that will be personally meaningful to *you,* at your local library.

I hope this chapter has helped you to accept your hearing impairment, given you an understanding of why you feel the way you do, and provided some helpful suggestions for coping with your social and emotional problems. I know that you're still going to have some anxieties, but now maybe you can view them more objectively and take some positive action for relieving them.

P.S. Incidentally, I was that girl with the crooked teeth whose story opened this chapter. I know my problem was minor compared with yours, but it did have a devastating effect on me at the time. I still have "horse teeth," by the way, but they don't keep me from smiling anymore. I hope you'll soon be able to say that about your hearing loss.

13

How can I find meaningful employment?

Blessed is the man that has found his work.—— Carlyle

I don't believe in the Puritan idea that hard work makes a person godly. Still, I do think that, for most of us, a feeling of *achievement* is essential to our sense of well-being. Anne Roe has indicated that work is probably the single most important activity in which individuals can seek to satisfy their psychological needs.[2]

If your hearing is impaired, you may be facing a career crisis. The characteristics of your personal crisis depend on the type and severity of your loss and your age at the time the loss occurred. You may have grown up in a school for the deaf, where you were trained for a specific job that has been phased out by modern technology. Or maybe you're not deaf, but have enough of a hearing loss that it's hard for you to keep up in regular college classes. Yet, you want to go into a field that demands higher education. Or maybe you've had normal hearing and a successful career for many years, but your hearing is failing now, and you're not sure you can continue in your present field. In any case, I think you'll find the suggestions in this chapter helpful if you have a job problem. It will contain some *guidelines*—

- for choosing the career that's best suited to your abilities, needs, and interests;
- for getting in touch with people and agencies that can help you;
- for locating the college, junior college, vocational technical school, or in-service training facility that can prepare you for your chosen occupation or for retraining in a new field;

- for *landing* that desired position;
- for success in *holding* the job.

First, let's look at some of the vocational trends that may affect your future.

What has been the success record of hearing-impaired people in employment? Hard-of-hearing and deaf people generally compare favorably with normally hearing workers in almost all fields of work, once they are given the chance. In fact, according to a national survey conducted by Lunde and Bigman, the deaf population reported a "higher average of earned income than its hearing counterpart."[2]

The deaf and hard of hearing have some special advantages over their hearing contemporaries. These include the fact that they usually show more concentration on the job because they aren't distracted by conversation and background noise. Also, depending on the *type* of hearing loss, they can sometimes work in noisy surroundings that would bother the normally hearing worker. (This is *not* the case, though, for those who have a problem with recruitment.) A Michigan Department of Labor report revealed the following facts:

> Workers with impaired hearing have a somewhat lower quit rate than unimpaired workers. The impaired lost about one day less in each 200 scheduled work days than unimpaired workers.
>
> Although disabling work injuries were more frequent among the impaired-hearing cases than among unimpaired workers, their injuries tended to be less severe.
>
> None of the injuries among unimpaired workers were attributed to a fellow worker's impairment.
>
> In none of the plants studied was any job re-engineering encountered for the workers with hearing defects. Although minor job modifications were made in some cases, it apparently had not been necessary to engage in any extensive job changes to utilize such workers.[3]

As I stated in Chapter 1, studies have shown conclusively that the deaf and hard of hearing have the same distribution of intelligence as those with normal hearing. It has also been demonstrated that hearing-impaired persons have the same capacities for abstract thought as do the nondeaf. Furthermore, deaf persons are equal to the hearing in manual dexterity and most other skills related to work. Their history until recent automation has been one of high rates of employment and stable job tenure.[4]

Still, unemployment is frequent among the hearing impaired, and many are working in jobs that are below the level of their abilities. And, you and I might as well face the facts. The technological advances of the past few years are creating a job squeeze that may hit the hearing handicapped pretty hard. For one thing, there's a shift, now, toward more white-collar jobs (accountants, engineers, scientists, teachers, and other professionals) and fewer blue-collar jobs (manual occupations, semiskilled and unskilled kinds of work). Then, too, the changing needs of technology sometimes make it necessary for people to be retrained for different types of work in midcareer. This retraining is more difficult for deaf persons than for hearing people. There is also a big increase in the number of jobs that require above-average language skills. And there's no doubt that educational requirements for employment are increasing.

That sounds pretty discouraging. Isn't there anything on the positive side? Yes. Most important, educational and training opportunities for the deaf and hard of hearing are increasing at a very fast pace (see Tables 1 and 2 later in this chapter); so the hearing impaired can be better equipped to compete. Also, more and more employers are hiring the hearing handicapped because they're finding out that these people are superior employees. In a recent survey of 480 major labor-market employers (that is, firms employing more than fifty persons), seventy-one percent of the employers indicated that they would have no objection to hiring deaf persons, but conditioned this by adding "if the applicants were qualified to perform the work." Furthermore, "approximately 85% who had employed deaf workers evaluated their performance as from good to excellent."[5] In addition to this, a tremendous increase—about fifty-one percent—is expected in service workers (practical nurses, hospital attendants, cooks, paraprofessionals, etc.). This is an area that offers excellent opportunities to the deaf and hard of hearing. Earl Klein points out that, "for the more able and advantaged of the deaf, enormous opportunities will exist in the professions and technical fields, and to a lesser extent in management and proprietary work."[6] E. Ross Stuckless has pointed out that "deafness itself does not preclude high levels of vocational attainment. There are very few professional classifications in which at least one deaf person cannot be identified."[7] Klein says, further, that "given good solid qualification, the deaf should be able to enter increasingly into a myriad of jobs, including many of those emerging from the new technology and the growing demand for services, where their handicap is either not a deterrent to satisfactory work performance, or rehabilitive steps can be taken to make an acceptable adjustment."[8] It seems obvious that more and better education and training are the keys that will unlock many of the doors that are closing now on the hard-of-hearing worker.

Is such training available for me? Yes. There are many federally supported training programs that can help you.

The Manpower Development and Training Act (MDTA) provides for both vocational education courses and on-the-job training. Check with your local state employment service office to see if you might qualify for assistance under this act.

The Social and Rehabilitation Service in the U.S. Department of Health, Education, and Welfare also helps in the rehabilitation and placement of persons with various types of handicaps, including hearing loss. The people in your local vocational rehabilitation office would be able to tell you what services you might obtain through this agency.[9]

If you're looking for a place to further your education or training, you may find the right facility for *you* in the following descriptive listing and tables prepared by Vernon and Snyder. I have the authors' permission to reproduce these here for your benefit.

> GRADUATE AND FOUR-YEAR COLLEGES. An increasing number of institutions of higher learning are providing supportive note-taking, interpreting, and tutorial services for deaf students. They are listed, here, described briefly, and then addresses are given of where to write for additional information.
>
> *Gallaudet College.* Gallaudet, the world's only college exclusively for the deaf, was established over 100 years ago. It offers study on the master's and undergraduate levels. In addition to extensive student services and on-campus housing accommodations, Gallaudet has a Preparatory Department where students of college potential who are not academically ready for college work are given a year of intensive advanced academic courses. For information, write Gallaudet College, Kendall Green, Washington, D.C. 20002.
>
> *National Technical Institute for the Deaf.* NTID offers study on the graduate (master's), undergraduate, and nondegree levels. It also provides on-campus housing and help in job placement. Major fields of study include business, science, engineering, art, photography, printing, and social work. Services for the students include interpreting, tutoring, note-taking aid, personal and medical counseling, and housing facilities. Both hearing and deaf students attend classes together, as the NTID is part of the Rochester Institute of Technology. For information, write NTID at Rochester Institute of Technology, 1 Lomb Memorial Drive, Rochester, New York 14623.

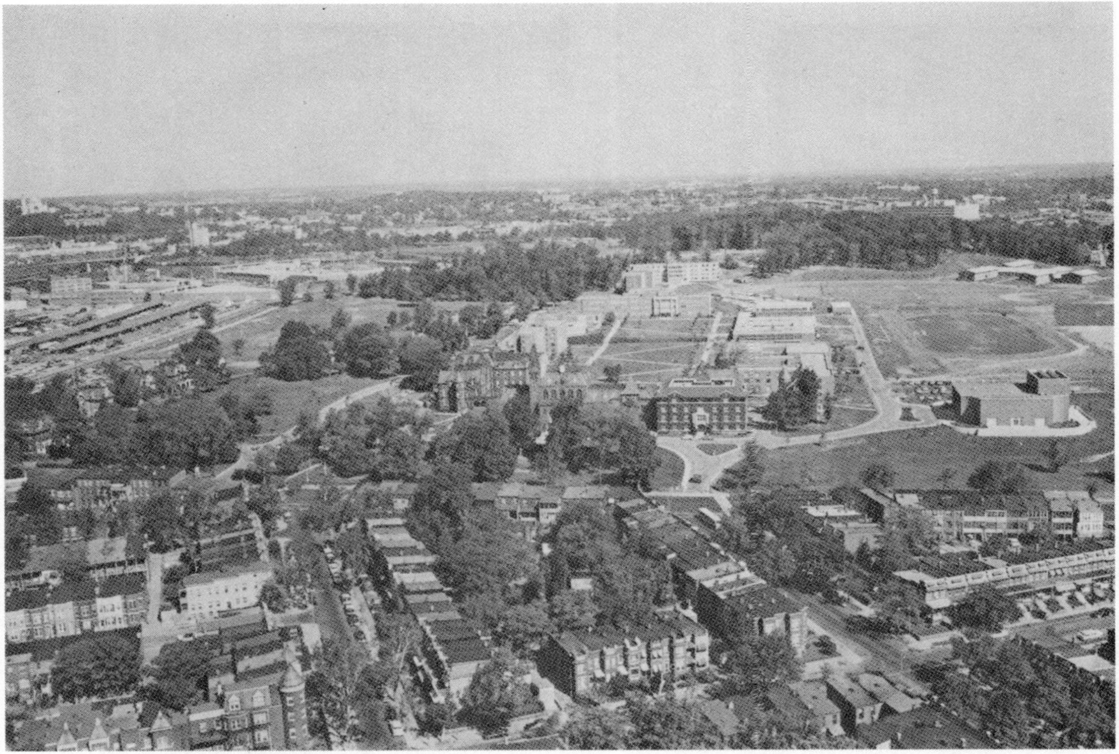

Figure 13.1. Aerial view of the Gallaudet campus. It is located in northeast Washington, D.C. (Gallaudet College photo.)

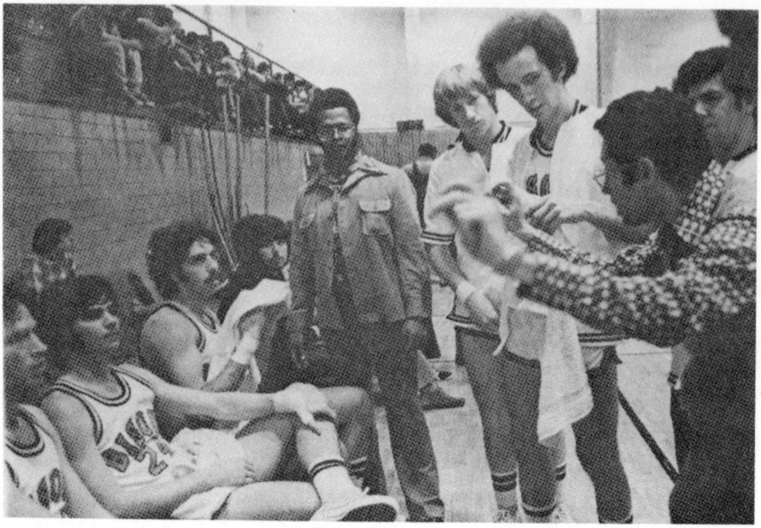

Figure 13.2. Gallaudet College fields teams in seventeen varsity sports and plays in the Potomac Intercollegiate Conference. (Callaudet College photo.)

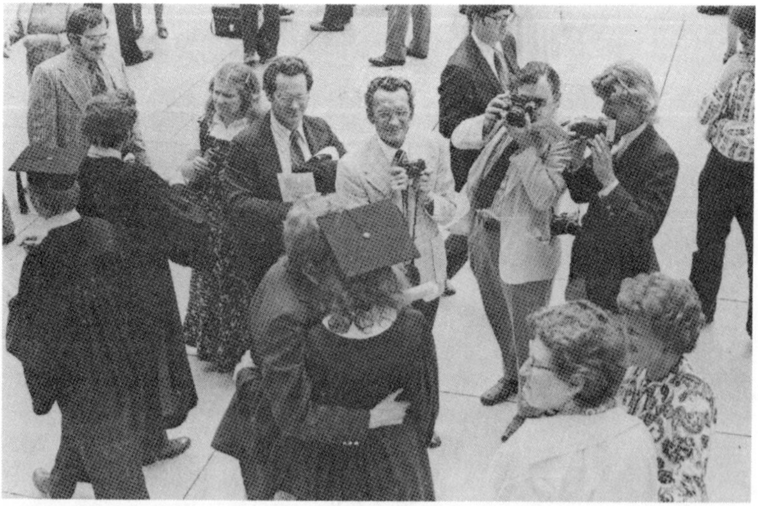

Figure 13.3. Commencement! (Gallaudet College photo.)

San Fernando Valley State College. The college offers educational programs on the graduate (master's) and undergraduate levels. Services to students include interpreting, tutoring, aid in note taking, and personal and medical counseling. Both on- and off-campus housing are available. For information, write College Services for the Deaf, Room 220, Engineering Building, San Fernando Valley State College, 18111 Nordhoff Street, Northridge, California 91324.

New York University. The university offers graduate training with programs clearly relating to the needs of the deaf students. Student services and housing are available. For information, write Deafness Research and Training Center, New York University, School of Education, 80 Washington Square East, New York, New York 10003.

University of Arizona. The university offers study for the Ph.D. and master's degrees, undergraduate work, and job placement. Student services include interpreting, tutoring, note-taking aid, physical therapy, personal and medical counseling, and dormitory facilities. For further information, write Department of Rehabilitation, College of Education, University of Arizona, Tucson, Arizona 85721.

University of Tennessee. The University of Tennessee is opening up many of its departments to deaf students. Services including interpreting and note taking are available through individual arrangements, and there is on-campus housing. For information, write the University of Tennessee, Department of Special Education and Rehabilitation, College of Education, Knoxville, Tennessee 37901.

University of Pittsburgh. Pittsburgh offers study on the graduate (Ph.D. and master's) level and placement services. Major fields of study include teacher education, rehabilitation, counseling, and special education. Services for deaf students include interpreting, tutoring, note-taking aid, and personal and medical counseling. For information, write University of Pittsburgh, Special Education and Rehabilitation, Bellefield Building, 160 North Craig Street, Pittsburgh, Pennsylvania 15213.

Central Bible College. The college provides a three-year training program to prepare deaf and hearing ministers for the deaf. Student services and housing are available. For information, write Central Bible College School for the Deaf, 3000 North Grant Street, Springfield, Missouri 65802.

Idaho State University. This university offers some graduate (master's) and undergraduate work, placement services, and a choice of vocational programs. Student services are limited but can include interpreting, tutoring, notetaking aid, personal and medical counseling, and on-campus housing. Inquiries should be directed to Director,

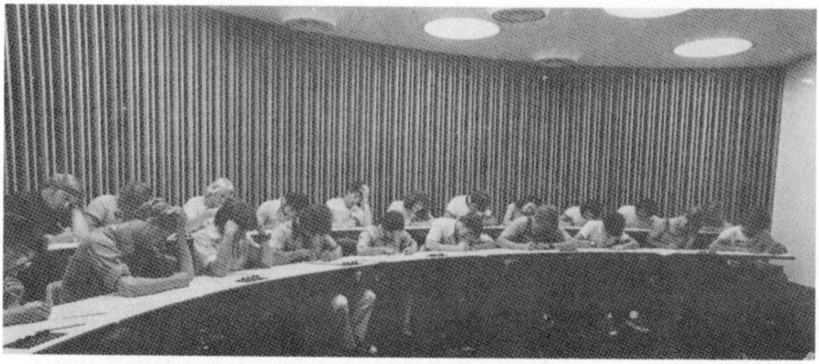

Figure 13.4. The cluster classroom at National Technical Institute for the Deaf offers a semicircular, tiered seating arrangement where students can benefit from the newest media and teaching techniques.

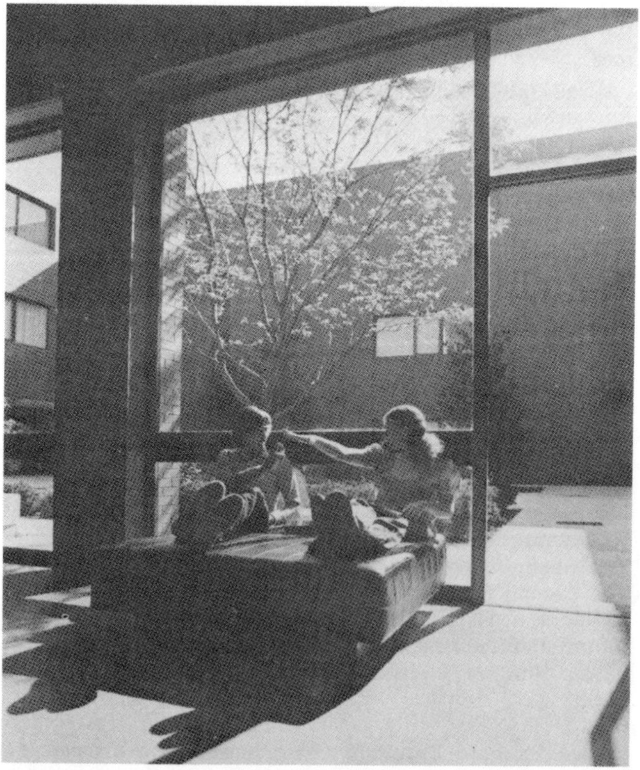

Figure 13.5. Two National Technical Institute for the Deaf students relax and chat between classes in the lobby of the NTID academic building.

Program Serving Deaf Students, Idaho State University, Pocatello, Idaho 83201.

JUNIOR COLLEGES AND VOCATIONAL-TECHNICAL SCHOOLS. A huge percentage of deaf youth qualify for and can benefit from junior college and vocational school education. In recognition of this, there has been a rapid increase in these kinds of programs. Basic information about these is given in Table 13.1. Some of these programs deserve specific mention. The St. Paul Vocational-Technical Institute is outstanding. It has the best of modern equipment and a large staff specialized in meeting the needs of deaf students. The Delgado and Seattle programs have similarly good staffs but not as extensive vocational course offerings.

The Hot Springs Rehabilitation Center serves multiply handicapped deaf persons. It is the only program in the world specifically created to serve these clients for whom the need is greatest.

Many of the programs listed in Table 13.1 will serve any deaf student in the United States, not just those in their locale. Also, many of the junior colleges and vocational schools take students with academic achievement scores as low as third grade. Perhaps 90% of deaf school leavers can benefit from one or more of the programs listed in Table 13.1, and they should be given every opportunity to attend.[10]

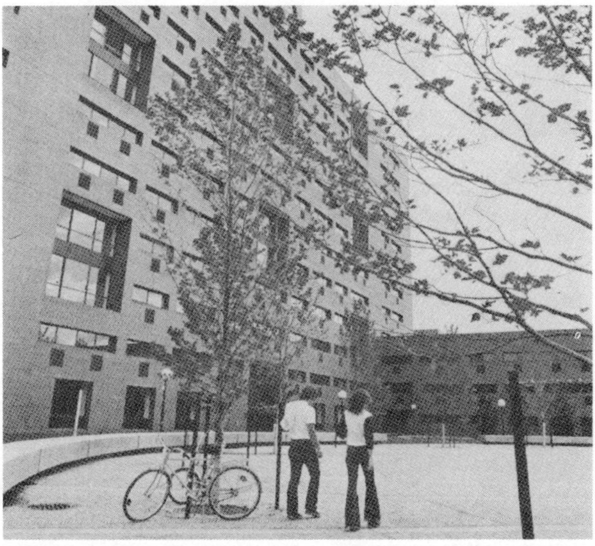

Figure 13.6. NTID students stroll through the courtyard in front of their twelve-story residence hall.

TABLE 13.1

Junior Colleges and Vocational Technical Schools Serving Deaf Students*
(All are coeducational)

● = yes; — = no.

Name and Address of Facility	Educational Programs: Placement Services	Educational Programs: Evaluation Services	Educational Programs: Assoc. of Arts Degree	Educational Programs: Average Length of Training Program	Admissions Requirements: Age Range	Admissions Requirements: Minimum Education	Admissions Requirements: Physical Limitations	Enrollment: Deaf	Enrollment: Hearing	Supportive Services: Interpreting	Supportive Services: Tutoring	Supportive Services: Note-Taking Aid	Supportive Services: Physical Therapy	Supportive Services: Personal Counseling	Supportive Services: Medical Counseling
Special Technical Facility P.O. Drawer 17 Fort Lashley Ave. Talladega, AL 35106.	●	●	—	2 yr	16+	open	ambulatory	70	200	●	●	●	—	●	●
Maricopa Technical College 106 East Washington St. Phoenix, AZ 85004.	●	●	●	2 yr	open	open	open	11	5000	●	●	●	—	●	—
Hot Springs Rehabilitation Center Hot Springs, AR 71901.	●	●	—	1 yr	16+	open	ambulatory no emotional problems	35	425	—	●	—	●	●	●
Golden West College 15744 Golden West St. Huntington Beach, CA 92647.	●	●	●	2 yr	18+	none	none	45	4000	●	●	●	—	●	—
Riverside City College 3650 Fairfax Ave. Riverside, CA 92506.	—	●	●	2 yr	17+	high school	none	30	5500	●	●	●	—	●	●
Community College of Denver Center for Hearing Impaired 1001 East 62nd Ave. Denver, CO 80216.	●	—	●	3 mo– 2 yr	18+	none	open	35	3000	●	●	●	—	●	—
American School for Deaf 139 North Main St. West Hartford, CT 06107.	●	●	—	1 yr	18–50+	3 yrs	ambulatory	240	none	●	●	—	—	●	—
Delgado College Program for Deaf 615 City Park Ave. New Orleans, LA 70119.	●	●	●	2½– 3 yr	18+	5 yrs	no mental, emotional, physical problems	70 to 75	4000	●	●	●	—	●	—
State Technical Institute and Rehabilitation Center Route 3 Plainwell, MI 49080.	●	●	—	1½– 2 yr	17½+	2 yrs and open	no mental illness	15+ 16 H of H	700	●	●	●	●	●	●
St. Paul Technical-Vocation Institute Tech. Voc. Prog. for Deaf Students 235 Marshall Ave. St. Paul, MN 55102.	●	●	DIPLOMA	1– 2 yr	17+	high school	none	c. 90	2000	●	●	●	—	●	●
Marie H. Katzenbach School for Deaf Sullivan Way West Trenton, NJ 08625.	●	●	—	3– 5 yr	16–21	none	IQ-65	150	none	●	●	—	—	●	●
Woodrow Wilson Rehab. Center Project for the Deaf Fisherville, VA 22939.	—	●	—	9– 12 mo	16–65	none	open	20	3	●	●	—	●	●	●
Seattle Community College 1625 Broadway Seattle, WA 98122.	●	●	●	1 yr	18+	4 yrs	emotional stability	75	10,000	●	●	●	—	●	—

*Since the writing of this article Harrison-Chilhowee Baptist Academy, Seymour Tennessee, has opened a college preparatory program specifically for deaf students. Brochures are available from the director, Edward Davis. The following schools also have programs for the deaf and information can be obtained by writing to them: St. Petersburg Junior College, Clearwater, Florida; Longbeach Junior College, Long Beach, California; Lee College (Junior College), Lee Drive, Baytown, Texas 77520.

What's Available for Deaf People

Services for Multihandi-capped	Living Accommodations					Costs				Financial Aid				Prep Program
	Board on Campus with Supervision	Aid Finding Off-Campus Housing	Student Makes Own Arrangements	Off-Campus Housing with Supervision	Commuters Only	Tuition and Fees	Room and Board	Transportation	Book Cost, etc.	Scholarships and Loans	Div. of Voc. Rehab. (D.V.R.) Aid	Direct Federal Fund	% on D.V.R.	
•	•	•	—	•	—		$350 mo covers all costs: is comprehensive			—	•	—	100	•
•	—	—	—	—	•	$20 up to 9 cr hrs. $40 over	—	private	$10 per class	•	•	•	80	—
•	•	•	—	•	—	$18 a day	—	—	vari-able	—	•	•	100	•
—	—	•	—	—	—	Free for residents, $30 per unit out-of-state		—	$75 per sem	•	•	—	60	•
—	—	•	—	—	—	—	$125 per mo	—	$50 per sem	—	•	—	100	—
•	•	—	—	—	—	—	$135 per mo	—	$40 per qtr	•	•	—	97	•
•	•	•	—	—	—		Approximate total costs: $4600 yr			—	•	—	95	—
—	—	•	—	•	—	$200 per sem	$120 per mo	$10 per mo	$75 per sem	—	•	•	100	•
							Out of State							
•	•	•	—	—	—	$288 $12 health fee	$200	—	$30	—	•	—	98	•
•	—	•	—	•	—	$670	$100 to $150 mo	—	$30 per sem	•	•	•	95	•
•	•	—	—	—	—	—	up to $10 per mo	—	—	—	—	—	—	•
•	•	—	—	—	—		varies				•	—	100	—
—	•	—	—	—	—	State $70 per qtr Out $170 per qtr	$975	varies	$100 per yr	•	•	—	90	•

(Reproduced by permission of McCay Vernon and Judith Ann Snyder)

TABLE 13.2—Evaluation Centers

• yes — no.

Name and Address of Facility	Admissions Requirements			Enrollment		Supportive Services						Services for Multi-handicapped
	Age Range	Minimum Education	Physical Limitations Accepted	Deaf	Hearing	Interpreting	Tutoring	Note-Taking Aid	Physical Therapy	Personal Counsel	Medical Counsel	
University of Arizona Rehabilitation Center Tucson, AZ 85721	Open	none	all accept.	17	25	•	—	•	•	•	•	•
Rehab Center for the Deaf P.O. Box 395 Cave Spring, GA 30124	15	none	open	200	none	•	•	—	—	—	—	•
Project for the Deaf Jewish Vocational Service One South Franklin St. Chicago, IL 60606	16	none	ambu-latory	100	5000	•	•	•	—	—	—	—
Res Prog for Speech & Hearing Impaired Young Adults Speech and Hearing Clinic Northern Illinois University DeKalb, IL 60115	16-24	none	open	65	none	•	•	•	—	—	•	•
Iowa State Vocational Rehab 1029 Des Moines Street Des Moines, IA 50300	16	none	open	4	70	•	—	—	•	—	—	•
Minneapolis Rehab Center 1900 Chicago Avenue Minneapolis, MN 55404	16-60	none	Dr's release	50	700	•	—	—	—	—	—	•
St. Paul Rehab Center 319 Eagle St. St. Paul, MN 55102	16	none	open	c6	100	—	•		•	•	•	•
Deaf Services, Work Exp Center of the Jewish Employment & Vocational Svc 2545 South Hanley Rd. St. Louis, MO 63144	16	none	ambu-latory	10	45 to 55	•	•	—	—	•	—	•
New York Society for Deaf Diagnostic Vocational Evaluation Center 344 East 14th Street New York, NY 10003	16	none	ambu-latory	35	none	•	•	—	—	•	—	•
Sunnyview Hospital & Rehab 1270 Belmont Ave. Schenectady, NY 12308	17	none	open	6	30	•	•	•	•	•	•	•
Pennsylvania Rehab Center 727 Goucher St. Johnstown, PA 15905	16	none	open	25	375	•	•	•	•	—	•	•
Wo Wilson Rehab Center Project for the Deaf Dept. Voc. Rehab Fisherville, VA 22939	15-65	none	open	4	25	•	•	—	•	•	•	•
West Va Rehab Center Institute, WV 25112	16	none	open	12	388	•	•	•	•	•	•	•
Wis. Sch. for Deaf Wis. Rehab Center for Deaf 309 Walworth Ave. Delavan, WI 53115	16-20	none	open	25 to 75	none	•	—	—	—	—	—	•

What's Available for Deaf People

Living Accommodations					Costs				Financial Aid			
Board on Campus with Supervision	Aid in Finding Off-Campus Housing	Off-Campus Housing with Supervision	Student Makes Own Arrangements	Commuters Only	Tuition and Fees	Room and Board	Transportation	Book Costs, etc.	Scholarships and Loans	Div. of Voc. Rehab. (D.V.R.) Aid	Direct Federal Funding	% on D.V.R.
—	—	—	—	•		Paid by D.V.R.			—	•	—	100
—	•	•	—	—		Paid by D.V.R.			—	•	—	100
—	—	—	•	•		D.V.R. Supported			—	•	•	80
•	—	—	—	—	$450	$270	—	—	—	•	—	99
•	—	—	—	—		D.V.R. Supported			—	•	—	?
—	•	•	—	—	$245 first wk	$45	$5 day	—	—	•	—	100
—	•	•	—	—		D.V.R. Supported			—	•	—	100
—	—	•	—	—	$50 wk	$130 mo	$6 wk first 2 wks only	—	—	•	—	100
—	•	—	—	—		D.V.R. Supported			—	•	—	100
—	•	—	—	—		D.V.R. Supported			—	•	—	90
•	—	—	—	•	varies	$6 day	—	—	—	•	—	100
•	—	—	—	—		varies		—	—	•	—	100
•	—	—	—	—	$18 day	$4 day	—	—	—	•	—	100
•	—	—	—	—		D.V.R. Supported				•	•	

Should I try to get a job on my own, or should I seek the help of rehabilitation agencies? The late G. Dewey Coats praised the job-getting ability of the hearing impaired. He stated: "Down through the years, the deaf as a group has written a credible record in gaining and holding jobs by their own efforts . . . and today, the great majority continue to land jobs with little or no help . . . but praiseworthy as this overall employment record is, I think many observers will agree that there are certain inherent disadvantages in the 'Do It Yourself,' sink or swim placement policy of past years."[11]

By seeking the help of a rehabilitation agency, especially if it's one that has counselors specially trained in working with the hearing impaired, you should get a thorough evaluation of your capabilities, interests, and potentials. These people know the job market and can act as a liaison for you in setting up interviews. They will give you expert individual attention and will follow through in helping you adjust to your job. Centers that specialize in the task of evaluating the hearing impaired are listed in Table 13.2, also prepared by Vernon and Snyder. If the centers listed here are not within traveling distance for you, check with your own state's vocational rehabilitation offices.

What other guidelines might help me to prepare for successful employment?

1. You would be wise to get training in broad skills rather than single specialties so that you can be more flexible in adjusting to the fast-changing job market.
2. Try to choose an occupation in which there is a critical demand for workers. Then get the best possible training in that area.
3. Explore the possibilities of on-the-job training.
4. Try to develop the personal qualities that employers seek. These include a strong sense of responsibility, maturity, dependability, punctuality, good judgment, flexibility, and the ability to get along well with others.
5. Learn how to properly fill out an application form.
6. Pay particular attention to good grooming.
7. If you've held previous jobs, get references from past employers.
8. Do not bring an interpreter with you for a job interview. As William Williams points out, "the deaf applicant who comes into an employment office with an interpreter naturally raises the question of what will happen when this employee tries to communicate on the job. Even if it means

pencil and pad, the deaf applicant should represent himself in the employment interview."[12]

9. Find out as much as you can about the prospective employer and his firm before you set up an interview.

10. Let the employer schedule the interview at his convenience. Never drop in unannounced.

11. Let him know when you ask for an interview (either by letter or, if you can communicate orally, by phone) that you do have a hearing problem.

12. If this employer has never had a deaf employee, be prepared to acquaint him with the highly successful work record achieved by deaf workers. It might help to take this book along and show him the answer to the question, "What has been the success record of hearing-impaired people in employment?"

13. Be prepared to make the employer aware of any special abilities you have that will help to compensate for your hearing loss. Most employers will choose a skilled or qualified deaf person in preference to an unprepared or unskilled hearing person any day. (If they don't, they need to have their heads examined!)

What pointers will help me to keep my job, once I've been hired? All of the things that help hearing people to hold their jobs, including—

1. willingness to follow direction,
2. a sincere interest in the company and its product(s) or service(s),
3. cooperation with fellow employees,
4. willingness to do extra work when necessary,
5. a minimum number of absences from work (always notify your employer when illness or other problems prevent you from going to work),
6. lack of bickering over petty differences in pay, job description, and status symbols.

You probably don't need to be reminded of these things, but remember that a good work record is *especially* important for you because you have to *prove* yourself, probably more than people without handicaps do. That may not be fair, but it's a fact you might as well face. Believe in yourself, and you can and *will* prove your worth. As Richard Sheridan said, "The surest way not to fail is to determine to succeed."[13]

No discussion of the employment future for the deaf would be complete without some reference to the advantages of *total communication.* Since the subject is chiefly of concern to parents and teachers of hard-of-hearing *children* and this is a book for hearing-impaired *adults,* we'll discuss it only briefly here.

What is total communication? There was a time, in the not-too-distant past, when many experts felt that children who were deaf or severely hard of hearing should be taught to communicate *only* orally. This idea was based on the belief that manual communication (fingerspelling and the language of signs) set deaf people apart from the hearing world. Of course, this is true to some extent. A person who cannot communicate orally is definitely handicapped in a hearing world. But there has been a change in the thinking of most professionals with regard to this matter. This change is based on two very important facts. First, experience with the oral method has proved that it is very difficult, if not impossible, to teach the profoundly deaf to communicate well enough orally to be understood satisfactorily. So children who were forced to rely on this method were *still* not able to communicate with the hearing. More important, carefully controlled studies have shown that children who were denied opportunity to learn and to use signing were seriously handicapped in their ability to learn. Their educational levels were far below the levels of their mental abilities, and this held true throughout the rest of their lives. Dr. Mervin Garretson, principal of the Model Secondary School for the Deaf, Washington, D.C., related the following anecdote, which can be applied to the deprivation suffered by deaf children who are forced into an oral-only method of communication:

> An elderly man in a large eastern metropolis became seriously ill and was rushed to a hospital where the diagnosis was quite bleak. It was felt that the old guy should be with relatives or close friends during what well might be his final days of life. It developed that he had no known living relatives and could give only one name—that of a boyhood friend, but he did not know his present whereabouts. The hospital staff decided to initiate a search for this unknown gentleman, practically combing the entire country. In time the man was located, flown to the city, and rushed to the hospital where he discovered his old friend under an oxygen tent. He hurried to his bedside to greet the dying man. The sick man tried to talk but words would not come. He waved feebly for a pencil and paper which were quickly given to him. Writing laboriously, he passed away with the paper

> still clutched in his hand. After the doctor had pronounced him dead, they pried the paper from his hand. He had scrawled: "Please get your foot off my oxygen hose."
>
> Thus, well-meaning but misinformed hearing authorities have held their collective foot on deaf children's communicative "hose," and figuratively killed their chances for an optimum education and a subsequently rich and rewarding life as self-sufficient and well adjusted deaf adults.[14]

The ability to understand the use of language (not speech, but words and their meanings) is basic to almost all areas of learning. Teachers of the deaf now realize that *any* means that can be employed to develop language concepts should be used as early as possible by deaf children, or they will never be able to catch up to the level of their abilities. Therefore, the emphasis, now, is on *total communication,* which takes advantage of *all* available means of language acquisition. A good definition of total communication is supplied by Margaret Kent, former principal of the Maryland School for the Deaf:

> . . . the right of a deaf child to use all forms of communication to develop language competence. This includes the full spectrum of child devised gestures, speech, formal signs, fingerspelling, speechreading, reading, and writing. To every deaf child should also be provided the opportunity to use any remnant of residual hearing he may have by employing the best possible electronic equipment for amplifying sound.[15]

Studies have shown that exposure to and use of manual communication does *not* interfere with oral speech development or lipreading skills.

As Vernon has observed, "Simply by the use of fingerspelling and the language of signs, academic gains, can, in general, be doubled or tripled."[16] The use of total communication, then, can greatly increase the educational achievement of the deaf and severely hard of hearing. Obviously, adequate education vastly improves their chances of finding employment in line with their intellectual abilities.

Should I learn manual communication as an adult? If you are planning to continue your education in one of the colleges or training institutions where total communication is used or at least understood, manual communication may increase your learning competency. Also, if you desire fellowship with other hearing-handicapped people, being able to communicate manually will help you to establish new and satisfying relationships.

Most important, though, since many deaf adults have hearing-impaired children, you should be aware of the advantages of the early use of total communication. If you have a deaf child, by all means learn the fingerspelling alphabet and the language of signs and *use* them in combination with speech as early as possible in your child's life. You will be giving him something worth far more than money or jewels.

Can I succeed in positions of high esteem if I'm deaf or have a severe hearing loss? Would you think a deaf person could be a highly successful actor? Teacher? Dentist? Clergyman? Counselor? Insurance man? Television actress or newscaster? Play director? Real estate manager? Psychologist? National executive director? Writer? Coach? President of a national society? The answer is Yes! to all of the above. A book published by the National Association of the Deaf recounts interviews with people who have reached high levels of attainment in all of these occupations. It's called *I'm Deaf, Too: 12 Deaf Americans*. It will give your morale a boost you may need. Write to: N.A.D., 814 Thayer Avenue, Silver Spring, MD, and request a copy, enclosing a check for $2.80.

Helen Keller's words are true for *you*: "We can do anything we want to do if we stick to it long enough."[17]

14

Where can I turn for help?

You are not alone. Helping hands are waiting to reach out to you from all directions. Many of the organizations and agencies that serve the hard-of-hearing population are run by people who are hearing impaired themselves. They know and understand your problems because they *share* them. But how can you accept their help if you don't know about them? In the previous chapter, we talked about colleges, training programs, and vocational rehabilitation services that can help you cope with your career problems. The purpose of this chapter is to acquaint you with other organizations, agencies, and publications that can help you in a variety of ways. Here is an alphabetical listing of these groups, with descriptions of the services they offer and addresses you can write to for more information.

Alexander Graham Bell Association for the Deaf, Inc., 3714 Volta Place, N.W., Washington, DC 20007. This is a nonprofit organization founded in 1890 by Alexander Graham Bell to encourage the teaching of speech, speechreading, and the use of residual hearing to the deaf. The association publishes *The Volta Review,* a journal that includes articles, book reviews, and news items on all aspects of hearing impairment. Send them a stamped, self-addressed envelope, and they'll send you their current book list, which offers works on all phases of hearing loss and includes price listings.

American Athletic Association of the Deaf, Inc., 3916 Lantern Drive, Silver Spring, MD 20902. The AAAD sanctions and promotes state, regional, and national basketball tournaments, softball tournaments, and word games for the deaf. Also, the AAAD sponsors AAAD Hall of Fame elections and the Outstanding Deaf Athlete of the Year award. The AAAD comprises 133 member clubs and approximately fifteen thousand individual members. Regional basketball tournaments are held in February and March each year. The *AAAD Bulletin,* reporting association affairs, is published quarterly.

American Speech-Language-Hearing Association, 10801 Rockville Pike, Rockville, MD 20852. This is a professional group whose members are trained to provide special services in speech, language, and hearing. It sets standards and certifies professional people working in the field. It can provide you with the name or names of a clinician or clinicians in your area who can help you with your speech and hearing problems. The association publishes the *Journal of Speech and Hearing Disorders* and the *Journal of Speech and Hearing Research.*

American Tinnitus Association, P.O. Box 5, Portland, OR 97207. This is a non-profit organization to aid tinnitus sufferers. Information and referral services are provided, as well as educational programs for the hearing professional.

Better Hearing Institute, 1430 K Street, N.W., Suite #600, Washington, DC 20005. This is "a non-profit educational organization providing public service, consumer education and public information programs for the hard-of-hearing, their families and friends.[1]

Board of Missions to the Deaf, The Lutheran Church—Missouri Synod, 500 North Broadway, Saint Louis, MO 63102. This organization is pledged to meet spiritual, moral, social, and cultural needs of the deaf and hearing handicapped. Under the direction of the Board of Missions, a staff of more than sixty full-time and part-time ministers and layworkers serve the deaf throughout North America and some foreign countries. Over five thousand adult communing members and about ten thousand baptized members are served in sixty-six congregations. Church services are conducted regularly in 267 additional cities in the United States and Canada. *The Deaf Lutheran* is the official monthly publication for the deaf of this organization.

The Canadian Association of the Deaf, 56A Wellesley Street, E., Toronto 284, Ontario. The goals of the CAD are similar to those of the National Association of the Deaf, but the organization for their accomplishment is somewhat different. An affiliate of this organization is the Canadian Deaf Information Center, which has a comprehensive collection of current books, periodicals, pamphlets, and clippings on deafness and the deaf. This collection is maintained in the form of a reference library open to the public.

Conference of Executives of American Schools for the Deaf, 5034 Wisconsin Avenue, N.W., Washington, DC 20016. This organization publishes the *American Annals of the Deaf,* in February, April, June, August, October, and December. The April issue is a directory of services for the deaf in the United States and includes a list of all teachers of the deaf.

Deaf Missions, Rural Route 2, Council Bluffs, IA 51501. This organization is interested in bringing Christ to deaf people. It offers Bible visuals, which consist of movies keyed with sign language and script, overhead transparencies, slide and film strips, and videotapes. Deaf Missions also maintains a comprehensive library of books and other printed literature about hearing loss. All of these materials are available for use by both hearing-handicapped individuals and those who work with them. Deaf Missions will mail them to you to use for two weeks. If you can afford a free-will offering for use of the materials, know that your aid will help make them available to those who can't afford to pay. You may want to write for the Deaf Missions catalog.

The Deafness Research Foundation, 366 Madison Avenue, New York, NY 10017. This foundation is organized to sponsor research into the causes and improved means of treatment and prevention of deafness and other ear disorders; to encourage young scientists to enter the field of otologic research; to sponsor a national public education program; to bring about a greater awareness of the seriousness of deafness; to urge regular ear examinations; and to encourage individuals with ear disorders to bequeath their inner ear structures to the Temporal Bone Bank Program for Ear Research. The foundation distributes a newsletter, *The Receiver,* several times annually.

Ephphatha Missions for the Deaf and Blind, The American Lutheran Church, P.O. Box 713, Sioux Falls, SD 57101. The Ephphatha Services Board has been commissioned to develop a climate of concern in every congregation of the American Lutheran Church for those who face life with a sensory impairment.

Episcopal Conference of the Deaf, 556 Zinnia Lane, Birmingham, AL 35215. This group is organized to promote and strengthen a ministry to the deaf in the United States within the Episcopal church. It is a union of missioners, clergy, and layworkers who, for the most part, are actively involved in working among the deaf in mis-

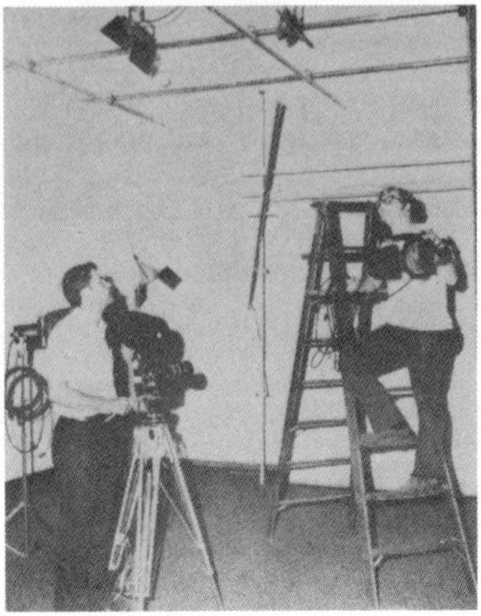

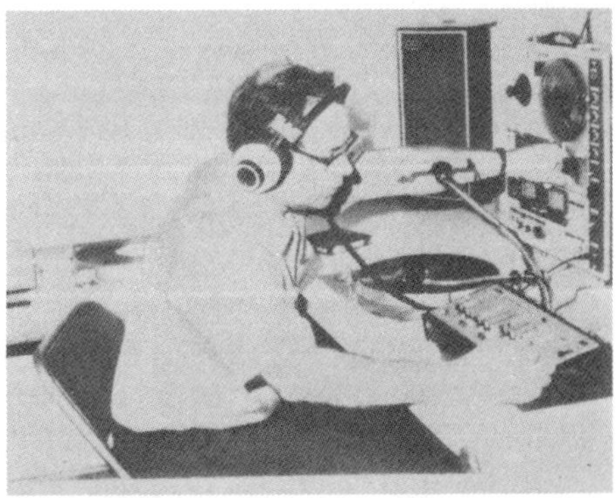

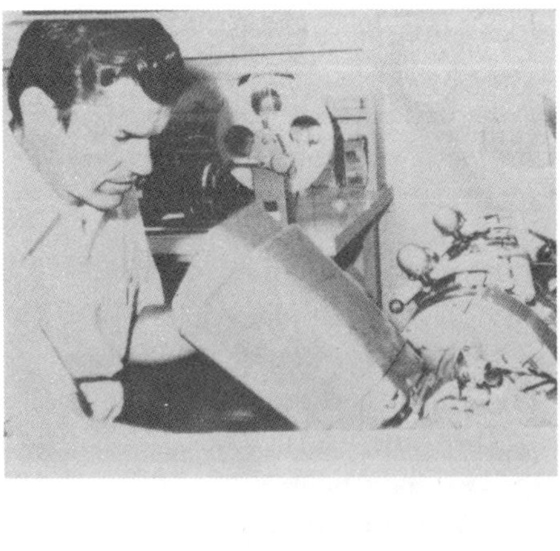

Figures 14.1, 14.2, and 14.3. Staff members at Deaf Missions, in Council Bluffs, Iowa, preparing filmed materials for the deaf.

sions and congregations. *The Deaf Churchman* is the official publication of the conference.

Gallaudet College Alumni Association, Kendall Green, Gallaudet College, Washington, DC 20002. As I mentioned in Chapter 13, Gallaudet is a college for the deaf. Its alumni association publishes the Gallaudet *Alumni Newsletter.*

Hearing Aid Manufacturers: A public service deserving special mention are the educational activities supported by the hearing aid industry. For instance, the Beltone Institute for Hearing Research publishes translations of scientific articles for distribution to professional workers in the field. Maico Hearing Instruments publishes an Audiological Library Series which is also for professionals in the field of audiology and otology. The Sonotone Corporation's publications include *Better Living* and other helpful pamphlets for those who use hearing aids. The Hearing Aid Division of the Zenith Radio Corporation supplies sound films for teaching purposes on request. Zenith also has a record entitled "Getting Through," which helps the family and friends of the hard of hearing to understand how speech sounds to the hearing handicapped.

International Catholic Deaf Association, 8419 Wesleyan Street, Vienna, CA 22180. This association is organized to promote a friendly and cultural bond of union among the Catholic deaf throughout the world, and to extend this union to members of other religious denominations; to be interested and actively engaged in all good works pertaining to the education and the social and ethical advancement of any deaf person. The association encourages the local chapters to arrange monthly communion masses in sign language. The chapters provide social, recreational, cultural, athletic, and religious programs for their own diocese. *The Deaf Catholic,* the official publication of the association, is issued bimonthly.

Mental Health Services for the Deaf, 1474 5th Avenue, San Francisco, CA 94143. This is a multipurpose, multidisciplinary center at the Langley Porter Neuropsychiatric Institute in San Francisco. In addition to conducting research, it supplies direct mental health services for deaf adults and children and their families. It also provides mental health consultation for agencies and professionals serving the deaf community. No fees are charged at this time.

National Association of the Deaf, 814 Thayer Avenue, Silver Spring, MD 20910. This is the only national civic organization run solely by and for the deaf. Its whole attention is directed toward ensuring that the rights and privileges of citizenship are maintained for the deaf. It serves as a clearinghouse; provides pamphlets, articles, and other information about the deaf; and will answer all inquiries concerning problems arising out of deafness. Its publications include: *Deaf American, NAD Newsletter,* and *Junior Deaf American.*

National Association for Hearing and Speech Action, 814 Thayer, Silver Spring, MD 20910. This association serves communicatively handicapped persons through about 170 community agencies that are members of NAHSA. NAHSA supplies information through television and radio spots, correspondence, workshop training sessions, a bimonthly magazine, a weekly publication called *Extracts,* and special pamphlets. In addition, NAHSA makes referrals to local service agencies, where they are available, for hearing tests, instruction in lipreading, auditory training, speech correction, assistance in the selection and use of hearing aids, instruction of preschool hearing-impaired children, and for speech problem diagnosis and treatment. NAHSA publishes a bimonthly magazine, *Hearing and Speech Action Magazine,* which is available on a subscription basis.

National Congress of Jewish Deaf, 6131 Claridge Drive, Riverside, CA 92506. This organization seeks to aid in the growth and preservation of the religious spirit of the Jewish deaf; to foster fellowship among them; and to maintain, for deaf Jews, the warmth and traditions of the Jewish home. The *NCJD Quarterly* is the official publication.

National Fraternal Society of the Deaf, 1300 W. Northwest Highway, Mount Prospect, IL 60056. This is a fraternal life insurance organization incorporated for the primary purpose of insuring deaf adults. The society, which operates on the lodge system, offers all standard forms of life insurance, accidental death benefits, waiver of premium benefits, and sickness and accident disability benefits. Membership in the society is open to all qualified adults, regardless of race, sex, or creed, who possess a hearing impairment.

New York State Mental Health Services for the Deaf. Outpatient psychiatric consultation and treatment are available here to deaf adults and older adolescents. A thirty-bed hospital ward serves those deaf adults and older adolescents who need psychiatric hospitalization. Finally, aftercare services, halfway-house facilities, and social and vocational rehabilitation are provided to patients in the various psychiatric programs. All means of communication are used—manual, oral, gesturing, and written.

Professional Rehabilitation Workers with the Adult Deaf, 814 Thayer Avenue, Silver Spring, MD 20910. The purpose of this organization is to encourage the development of a better understanding of the needs and problems of the deaf. *The Journal of the Rehabilitation of the Deaf* is the official publication of PRWAD.

Psychosomatic and Psychiatric Institute of Michael Reese Hospital, 3033 S. Cottage Grove Avenue, Chicago, IL 60608. At present, outpatient care is offered here on a limited basis. Psychiatrists in private practice who are experienced in working with deaf patients are affiliated with this institute.

Registry of Interpreters for the Deaf, P.O. Box 1339, Washington, DC 20013. The registry has a total membership close to two thousand. It publishes a directory of its members, which is updated annually. If you need an interpreter, write to this organization.

Saint Elizabeth's Hospital—The Mental Health Program for the Deaf, 2700 M. L. King Avenue, Washington, D.C. 20032, is designed to provide comprehensive mental health services for the deaf and mentally ill. It includes inpatient and outpatient care, partial hospitalization, and twenty-four-hour-a-day emergency services. Anyone desiring to help a deaf person who is having mental problems might do well to first contact Saint Elizabeth's, which can accept a patient from anywhere in the United States or refer him to facilities in his own locality.

These are some of the major organizations and agencies serving the hearing handicapped. Maybe one or more of them will be able to help you with some of the special needs that you have. Feel free to write to the above addresses for further information. For a more complete listing, get a copy of the April issue of *American Annals of the Deaf.*[2]

In addition to national groups, check to see if there are any local organizations in your community that can provide you with services or just offer fellowship with others who share your problem. Call your local chamber of commerce.

As you can see from this listing, the statement I made at the beginning of the chapter really is true: *You are not alone.*

15

What can my family and friends do to help me and to cope with the problems my handicap creates for them?

"I'm worried about Joe. He used to be so good natured, but now he seems depressed all the time. He snaps at the children, accuses me of mumbling, and retreats to the bedroom whenever company comes. His hearing loss is a big strain on the whole family." Mrs. Brown (name changed) sat across the desk from me, twisting her handkerchief as her husband stared at the floor.

"Mary just doesn't understand. She says I ignore her, but it's just that she mumbles all the time. And the kids! They laugh at me when I try to get into the conversation because half the time I blurt out something that is way off the subject. People are always turning down the TV in the middle of my favorite programs, and when friends come over, they often shout at me or treat me like a child. That hurts!"

Like vinegar poured into milk, hearing loss can sour family relationships. But it doesn't *have* to be that way! Here are some answers that may improve the flavor of your family life.

Why won't my husband listen to me? I can shout until I'm blue in the face, but he just turns me off. Many people with impaired hearing, especially those with sensori-neural losses, have a low threshold of pain. This means that loud noises hurt their ears, even more so than for people with normal hearing. Besides, most people with such losses have no trouble hearing *voices,* which fall mostly in the low and middle frequencies. It's the high-frequency consonant sounds that they can't hear, and this is why your husband can hear your normal voice and still not be able to understand what you're saying. Shouting doesn't help. It hurts. So instead of raising your voice, touch his arm to get his attention and wait until he is looking at you. Then speak slowly and distinctly.

Should I lean forward and speak directly into his ear or hearing aid microphone? No. This makes him self-conscious, and, if you do it in public, it embarrasses him by calling attention to his handicap.[1] Then, too, the volume control on his aid is set for conversation at normal distances, and your action may cause him physical discomfort.

Should I have my dad face the window when I talk to him, so that he can see better? Good lighting is essential to good lipreading, but the light should be on *your* face, not his. Have the source of light behind him while you sit or stand in front of him. That way, your facial features will show up clearly, and the light will not get in your father's eyes and impair his ability to see what his ears miss. This may seem to be a nuisance at first, but if you get in the habit of paying attention to the light source, you'll soon find yourself doing it automatically.

Should I exaggerate my lip movements when speaking to him? Definitely not. This seems to be the natural thing to do, but it only makes understanding more difficult for him because you are distorting words. His hearing loss has caused him to be very alert to the way normal speech sounds *look,* but when you exaggerate your speech movements, you actually interfere with his lipreading ability. And can you imagine how these contortions make *you* look, and how they make *him* feel?

What else can I do to make lipreading easier for him? Look directly at him when you speak. Don't try to talk to him while his back is turned. Keep your head and body still while you're speaking except for the normal gestures you use. Your hand and arm movements give him clues about what you're saying, but if you keep changing body positions, he'll have trouble following your lip movements. "If you sit in a rocking chair, *do not* rock back and forth while talking! Consider the listener; if you must rock for your own comfort, he is forced to follow your motions to and fro in order to catch the visible movements of speech. This is an exhausting ordeal that the hard-of-hearing person could be spared with a little sacrifice and self-control on your part."[2] Have you ever tried to read the newspaper while someone else is holding it? Every time he moves, you lose your place. That's how the lipreader feels when you keep moving as you're talking to him.

Don't talk with your mouth full. You can't help chewing while talking; so your lip movement is distorted. (Besides, who wants to look at *that,* in order to "hear"?) If you chew gum, take it out when you talk to your father, (even if you have to stick it on the end of your nose!) Don't try to talk to him while holding a cigarette, cigar, or pipe between your lips. A bright shade of lipstick will help make lip movements plainer, too. Remind your husband that his mustache makes it harder for your father to understand him. Improving in-law relations may be worth a shave.

How can I get my wife to wear her new hearing aid? First read Chapter 8, so that you will be aware of the gradual process that she needs to follow in adapting to her new aid. Remember that this appliance cannot give back your wife's hearing. It's only a tool and an imperfect one at that. She'll have to experiment and practice before she will be able to use it to best advantage. This requires patience on her part and on yours. Try to understand the annoyance and frustration she feels, and keep expressing your confidence in her ability to overcome the tribulations she endures while she learns to use it. Never be overpersistent about the use of the aid. Encourage but don't nag, and she'll eventually achieve success in adjusting to this valuable piece of equipment.

I bought my wife an expensive hearing aid, but she still says "what?" and "huh?" All the time. Why? Again, remember that a hearing aid is not a miracle. It's just the best we have. It *aids,* but does not *restore* natural hearing. You still need to speak slowly and distinctly and to make sure she can see your face when you talk to her. And there may be another reason for the whats and huhs. She may be so used to not hearing that these responses are habitual. Once in a while, reply to "what?" by asking sympathetically, "What do you think I said?" You may both be surprised to find that she really did hear you after all, and the habit will soon disappear.

I get so tired of repeating the same sentence over and over. Is there a better way? If your hard-of-hearing husband doesn't understand what you've said, rephrase your sentence. Say it another way. Suppose you've asked, "Are you ready to eat?" and he comes back with, "Turn down the heat?" Don't laugh or become impatient. Say, "Dinner's ready. Come to the table." Or, "We're having chicken for dinner. Can you come now?" You have saved him from embarrassment and prevented some frayed nerves for both of you.

But what if I reword my sentence and he still misunderstands? Keep pencil and paper handy. Write down key words, and after he has read them, repeat your message so he can see it on your lips. This will help him improve his lipreading ability. Lipreading is a tough job that requires lots of practice. The paper-and-pencil technique will help, because he sees the words first in writing, then on your lips.

My hard-of-hearing wife has very poor speech, and I often have

trouble understanding her. What can I do about this? It will help if you watch her face intently as she speaks. *She* picks up clues through facial expression and lipreading, and you can, too. Be very careful not to show signs of annoyance. This will be difficult sometimes, but remember that hard-of-hearing people are extra sensitive to the reactions of others. She desperately *wants* to be understood, so don't *blame* her for not speaking clearly. Just calmly ask her to "please repeat that slowly," and keep a smile in your eyes. If this is a *frequent* problem for the two of you, suggest that she carry a pencil and paper.

My deaf uncle has come to live with us. Should we use manual communication (sign language) with him? The answer to this question depends upon many factors. If his hearing loss occurred when he was a very young child, before he had a chance to develop oral language, he is probably already using manual communication. By all means, make sure that every member of your family learns to sign, so that you can all communicate with your uncle.

If, however, his hearing loss occurred later in life and is not severe enough to interfere drastically with his ability to communicate, it's probably better to stay with oral communication. Otherwise, he may come to rely so much on signing that he stops trying to communicate orally, and this will obviously limit the number of people with whom he has relationships.

On the other hand, if his hearing is impaired to the point that it is no longer usable for communication, and his lipreading ability is meager, then you and he have nothing to lose and a great deal to gain by learning manual communication. It's better to be able to converse easily with a few close associates than to be completely cut off from the social interaction that language (even silent language) makes possible. Friends and coworkers can also learn to sign in order to get ideas across quickly and accurately to deaf persons.

There are basically two types of manual communication: fingerspelling (which uses a different finger position for each letter of the alphabet) and signing (which uses standardized gestures to represent whole words or concepts). You will probably want to use a combination of both. Many fine books are available for learning the language of signs. One of the best is *Signing Exact English,* by Gustason, Pfetzing, and Zawolkow.

It is best, if possible, to use the "simultaneous method," in which the speaker talks and spells or signs at the same time. This is faster than writing out ideas and messages on a blackboard or pad and paper, and, most important, it keeps those communication lines open.

Why is my husband rude to guests? When we have a group in, he often just goes off into the bedroom when the evening is only half over. It is important for you to realize that a hard-of-hearing person can take only so much confusion and group noise. He doesn't mean to be rude, but social gatherings become a real strain for him after a while, and he really *needs* to retreat to a quiet place in order to keep his nervous and emotional balance.

You should also consider the fact that, while you feel that your husband has been rude to the guests, he may feel that they have been rude to him. It's very easy for a group of normally hearing friends or relatives to get so involved in their repartee, small talk, and spontaneous laughter that they forget all about the hard-of-hearing person who is sitting there feeling stranded. How would you feel if you were at a party where everyone spoke a language you couldn't understand and no one bothered to interpret for you? Would you want to sit there all evening? You can help your husband to feel more a part of things if you occasionally make it a special point to fill him in on the subject of the conversation. "Aunt Ethel is telling about her operation," or "Did you know that Ted and Jane are taking a trip to Europe?" As the conversation shifts to a new topic, give him a clue so he can follow along. Get in the habit of showing him, by a simple hand gesture, when the conversation moves from one speaker to another.

Another thing you can do to help is to get him involved as a host. Suggest that he serve the drinks. If he loses the train of conversation, he can circulate about refilling glasses or pouring coffee and still feel a part of the group.

It's probably best to invite only one or two friends in at a time. Your husband is more likely to maintain his sociability that way.

My wife is getting to be paranoid. She thinks everyone is talking about her all the time. This, too, is a natural reaction. We all have a little of this in us, especially when people are whispering in our presence. Just make sure you never say anything in your wife's presence that you don't intend for her to hear. Speak *to* her, not *about* her. Some people discuss problems relating to their hard-of-hearing relatives while they're in the same room, by covering their mouths with their hands. This is deliberately taking advantage of the person's poor hearing, and that's hitting below the belt.

Why does my wife's hearing seem to get worse at night? Well, there's the obvious reason of poorer lighting, which makes lipreading more difficult. But there may be another factor involved. Most hard-of-hearing people are plagued by tinnitus, intermittent or constant head noises (ringing in the ears). She has to listen *through* these annoying noises, which often increase in intensity when she's tired or depleted nervously.[3] Many hearing-handicapped people require a great deal of sleep because they are under a constant strain. Encourage your wife to take a nap in the afternoon, and be understanding if she needs to go to bed early at night.

Why does grandpa snap at the children for no reason at all? He doesn't do it "for no reason at all." He gets annoyed with them for several very logical reasons. For one thing, they often startle him by bursting in on him when he's alone or by touching him unexpectedly. Teach them to approach him from the front, so that he can see them coming, or, if they do come from behind, have them give a short, sharp tap on the floor when they're still a few feet away. The vibration will alert him to their presence. Children also have a tendency to laugh at the communication errors hard-of-hearing people make, and if you've ever been made fun of by a child, you can understand why grandpa snaps. It's a big fat jab in the ego. Talk to the kids. Remind them of some time when their friends made fun of them. Help them remember how it felt. Appeal to their pride in being grown up enough not to hurt grandpa's feelings. They'll come around, and when they do, they will have soaked up one of the most important human values they'll ever learn—the ability to feel compassion. Children are by nature noisy, and noise hurts grandpa's ears and makes his nerves scream. So *he* screams. It's not fair to the children to go around shushing them all the time, but they *can* learn to do their noisy playing and "fighting" outside, or in the basement, or someplace where grandpa *isn't.* Don't segregate the children from their grandfather, though. There are lots of things they can enjoy together, such as watching TV, working on jigsaw puzzles, building models, and playing card games. Hard-of-hearing people want and need companionship, and grandpa and the kids can become real pals, if they build the right kind of bridge.

My husband and I were glad to have mother move in with us, but she's beginning to get on my nerves. She just sits around all day feeling sorry for herself. Maybe she feels unneeded. One thing we all need is a feeling of accomplishment. Encourage your mother to help around the house. Ask her to do special favors for you, then let her know how much you appreciate her help. Try to interest her in learning to do something she's never done before. Does she know how to type? If not, get her a typewriter and a self-teaching manual. Developing a new skill will build up her confidence, and typing can also help to fill in an occasional communication gap. Maybe she'd like to become a contest buff. Lots of people enter contests as a hobby, and there's even a magazine she can subscribe to that will keep her informed about current contest offerings. Just think what winning would do for her ailing ego! You know her well enough to think of hobbies that would appeal to her and special abilities she could develop that don't require good hearing. If she resists one thing, try another. It may be an effort on your part at first, but anything you can do to pull her out of that stagnant pond of self-pity will be well worth your time. Encourage her to follow the suggestions in Chapter 12 for improving her emotional outlook on life.

Why is it so hard for my husband to talk on the telephone? For one thing, he can't lipread over the phone. Also, some callers neglect to speak directly into the mouthpiece, so his hearing problems are intensified. Many mechanical devices are available to help with this problem. Your local phone company can install a special hard-of-hearing telephone with a volume control knob in the receiver. You can turn it down when you talk; your husband can turn it up. A bone conduction receiver is available for people with severe conductive losses, and you can also get a device that allows a third person to "plug in" on a conversation. Using this appliance, you can repeat

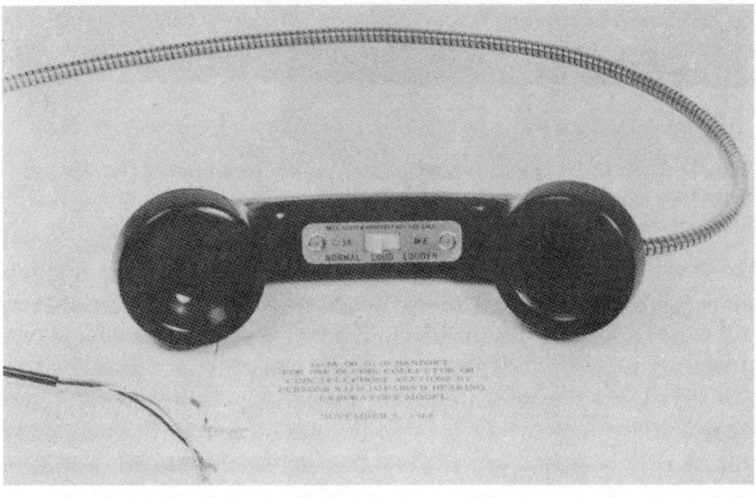

Figure 15.1. It is easy to adjust the level of loudness with a telephone receiver such as this one. (Photo courtesy of American Telephone and Telegraph.)

what the caller says, and your husband, having read your lips, can carry on his side of the conversation on his own. Or, to go another route, several models of hearing aids have a specially designed "telephone pickup." The user just flips a switch on his aid and holds the telephone receiver against the case of his instrument. If you're planning on getting a new phone, you need to be aware of the fact that some types of telephones—Trimline and some of the unusually styled phones in the Design Line—won't work with hearing aids. To transmit sound to a hearing aid, these phones have to be used with a special adapter. The adapters can be purchased from hearing aid firms or the phone company.

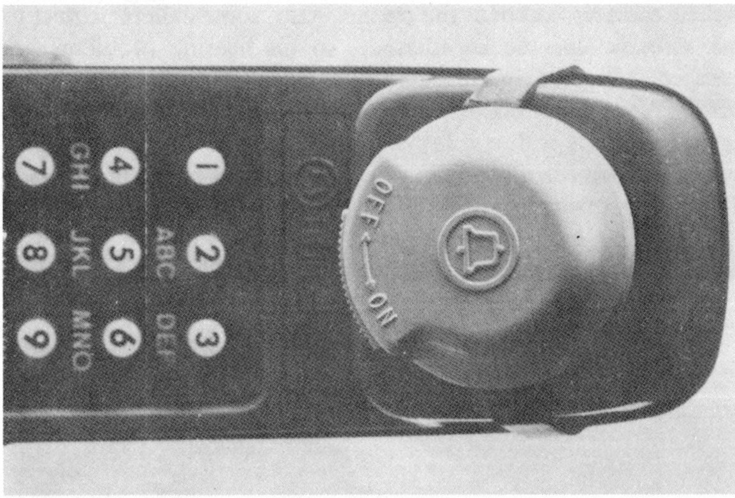

Figure 15.2. An adapter for increasing loudness fits on the receiver of Trimline and Design Line telephones for use by the hard of hearing. (Photo courtesy of American Telephone and Telegraph.)

These should make talking on the phone much easier for my husband, but how can he tell when the phone is ringing? There are several ways of solving this problem, depending on the degree and type of hearing loss. The telephone company can provide a louder signal or a signal in a different frequency range. A person who can't hear the usual telephone ringing signal because of a high-frequency loss may be able to hear a low-pitched buzzing sound instead. The standard telephone can be equipped with any one of six different frequency ranges at no extra cost. A horn or a large gong can also be hooked up to the phone (if your neighbors are far enough away!). Or

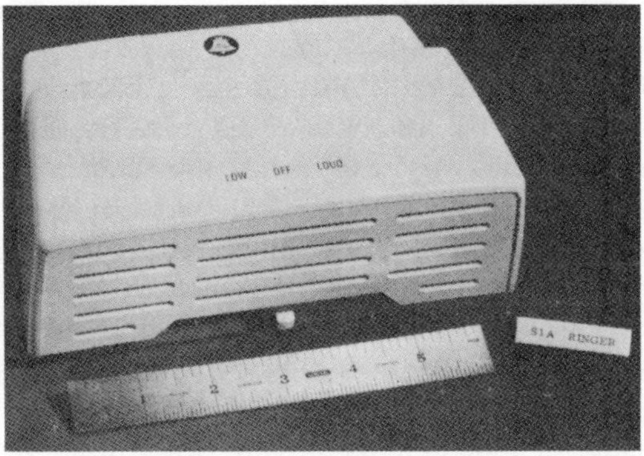

Figure 15.3. Telephone signaling devices, such as the above Tone Ringer, make it possible for hearing-impaired people to know when someone is calling. (Photograph courtesy of American Telephone and Telegraph.)

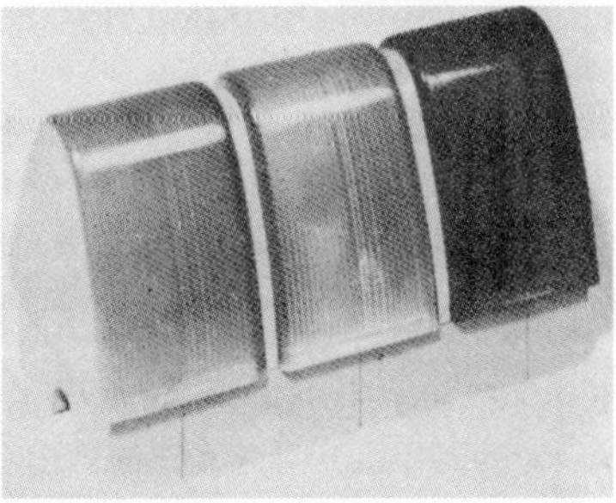

Figure 15.4. Lamp indicators light up to signal that the phone is ringing. (Photo courtesy of American Telephone and Telegraph.)

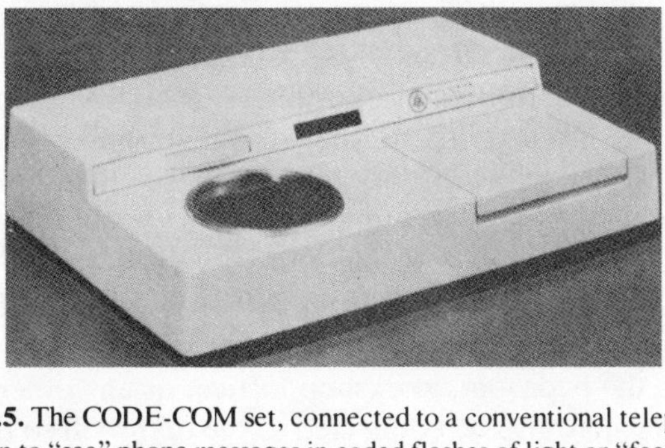

Figure 15.5. The CODE-COM set, connected to a conventional telephone, allows a deaf person to "see" phone messages in coded flashes of light or "feel" them in the vibrations of a finger pad. Light flashes come from a recess (black rectangle) in the center of the raised portion of the set. The circular vibrating pad is on the left. The sending key on the right, used like a telegraph key, is for deaf people without speech. If the deaf person can talk, he speaks into the telephone handset in the normal manner. (Photo courtesy of American Telephone and Telegraph.)

you can get an "auxiliary signal control device" that causes a light to flash or a fan to blow when the phone rings. Check with your telephone company for details about these conveniences.

What can we do about the problem of TV? Dad turns it up so loud it about drives the rest of us out of the house, but if we turn it down, he can't hear it. Check with your local TV and radio stores. They can order him a set of headphones, with built-in volume controls, for listening to TV, radio, and the phonograph. For this purpose, the headphones usually give far better results than hearing aids. Or, your hearing aid dealer may be able to provide him with an inexpensive device called an *inductor,* to be used with a hearing aid. This device substantially improves the clarity of television, radio, and record player reception for the hearing handicapped. Why not get one of these devices for your father for his birthday? It'll be a present for the whole family!

My wife can't hear the baby when he cries. She has to check on him every few minutes, and this is making her a nervous wreck. You can install an intercom system that picks up sounds in one room, such as the nursery, and delivers them, amplified, to another, such as the kitchen or bedroom.

Grandpa likes to keep his door locked. How can we wake him at the proper time? You can get a light-flashing alarm clock if he's not a heavy sleeper, or an electric vibrator connected to a timer and placed under the mattress will awaken him at the right time. Or, to save money, use a little ingenuity. Attach a long string to his wrist and extend it under the door. A good tug from the outside, repeated if necessary, is sure to wake the soundest sleeper![4]

If he spends a lot of time in his room and you want to get his attention while he's awake, "use a long string run under the door or through the keyhole, with a bit of crumpled paper tied to the end."[5] Place the paper end where Grandpa can see it. A pull on the other end indicates that someone is at the door.

How can I get my husband's attention when he's in the basement and I'm upstairs? Signal lights that flash when a button is pressed can be installed in the bedroom, workshop, office, or any other room in the house. They may also be connected to the door bell so that lights flash in several places at once when the door bell rings.

Why does Uncle John get so mad when I tell him it's better to be deaf than blind? *Is* it? How do you know? Because a blind man must also subsitute one sense for another, blindness and deafness are often classed together, but they are two completely different problems.

There really is no adequate way to compare them except to say that whichever handicap you have is worse as far as you're concerned. When you tell Uncle John that it's better to be deaf than blind, he resents the belittling implication. If you're blind, then the two of you can have a rousing debate about it, but if you're not, then you have no basis for your statement. You need to recognize the fact that deaf people face some anguishing problems from which the blind are spared. (Of course, the reverse is true, too, but we're talking about *Uncle John's* problem now.) For one thing, blindness is usually apparent to any observer. The deaf person's handicap often goes unnoticed unless he is spoken to, because he has no distinguishing visible feature that shows him to be other than a normally hearing person. In fact, strangers often mistakenly consider him retarded because of the blank, uncomprehending look on his face when they speak to him. I know one man who is almost totally deaf, but who wears a hearing aid even though it doesn't help his hearing, just so people will know that he's deaf and not mentally incompetent. When Uncle John talks about his problems, listen and sympathize instead of telling him he's lucky not to have some other handicap.

Should I give my hard-of-hearing wife advice about her hearing problem? You may want to make suggestions, now and then, but be careful not to push. Most people resent being told what they *should* do, especially if they haven't asked for advice, and hearing-impaired people are no exception. The best way to help your wife is to make sure she has the best professional help available. Go with her to see the otologist, the audiologist, the speech and hearing clinician, and the hearing aid dealer. Let them give the advice.

What if she *wants* to talk to me about her hearing problem? Then be available and be a good listener. There's a little technique used by counselors that's called "active listening." As your wife talks about her problems, listen for the *feelings* she's trying to express. Then, instead of giving advice, let her know you understand how she feels. For instance, she might say, "I just wish Mrs. Jones wouldn't shout at me when we're at church circle. Doesn't she know I wear a hearing aid and read lips?"

You might be tempted to say, "Well, after all, you're hard of hearing. You're just going to have to learn to put up with that sort of thing." That will only make your wife feel worse. Instead, say, "It must really be embarrassing to have people shout at you in public. I suppose it makes you feel like crawling in a hole." If you get in the habit of responding this way, she'll be able to get her feelings out in the open instead of letting them smolder inside of her. She doesn't really want advice. She just wants to know that someone understands her hurt feelings. She'll be able to carry her hearing-loss burden as long as she knows you're walking beside her, instead of pushing or pulling.

Sometimes I think my husband is just being difficult or lazy. Couldn't he hear better if he'd just make more effort? "Probably no one but the hard-of-hearing person himself fully understands the mental and emotional strain caused by loss of hearing."[6] True, there are people who don't hear because they won't. But we're talking about one whose hearing is genuinely and severely impaired. I'd suggest that you try wearing a good, tight-fitting pair of ear plugs for a day. Don't cheat by taking them out to answer the phone or run to the store or chat with your neighbor. By nighttime, you may have a better concept of some of the problems your husband struggles with every minute of every day.

Those of us who have normal hearing take it so much for granted! I always ask my beginning audiology students to make a list of the ways in which they use their hearing during a twenty-four hour period. Why don't you try this, too? You'll probably find yourself listing such things as: knowing when the toast pops up without having to look, feeling the warm glow that a compliment brings, enjoying the sermon in church, hearing the laughter of your children, the sound of rain on the roof, relaxing to music, enjoying a movie, hearing the birds sing. . . . What a lot of living you would miss, what a huge chunk of life would be taken from you, if you lost your hearing! Think about it.

What else can I do to help? Try to learn as much as you can about your loved one's hearing impairment. Read *all* the chapters in this book, and discuss them with him. Be his "family helper" for practice in lipreading, auditory training, and speech conservation and training.

A little extra patience, understanding, and ingenuity will make family life easier for you and for the hard-of-hearing person you love. Remember that he is not his hearing loss. He is a normal human being with an imperfection. What's yours?

Most important of all, let him know, in little ways and big ways, that you love him just the way he is.

16

What does the future hold for me?

As I sit here this morning,
writing the final chapter in my book
for you, hundreds of scientists, researchers,
and engineers around the world are investing their
hours and their hearts in your future. At last the hearing-impaired population, so long a neglected minority, is beginning to reap some of the fruits of our advanced technology, innovative medical procedures, and creative educational advances.

So what's new? The last few years have brought remarkable progress in hearing aid design, and it is reasonable to expect better quality of sound transmission, increased durability, and improved hearing aid design in the future. Canfield notes that batteries are no longer needed for some experimental aids that are worn in sunlight and solar powered, and he speculates that, "if this limitless power can be channeled into the ear to stimulate the delicate mechanism that sends signals to the brain, who knows what may come next?"[1]

A recent newspaper article reported that hearing aid makers are developing an aid small enough to be buried in the flesh of the ear, and equipped with the same long-lasting batteries used in heart pacemakers. The device can be transplanted into the ear by an operation and changed only once every five years.

At West Virginia University, electrical engineering students are cooperating with speech therapists on a device that allows severely hard-of-hearing people to "see" voices.[2] It helps the deaf to adjust pitch and loudness so that their voice quality is more nearly normal. Is it too much to hope that perhaps someday such an instrument could be refined to the point that it could be used as a visual means of understanding speech?

About two thousand deaf families in the United States now own teletypewriters, which allow them to carry on telephone conversations without hearing. Lee Brody, a deaf real estate manager and president of the New York–New Jersey TTY for the Deaf, Inc., tells us of some new developments in this area:

> We have a new TTY that you can take with you, anywhere you go. It has no motor. It is light and small enough to fit into a briefcase.
>
> Another new TTY hooks onto T.V. sets. The messages appear on the T.V. screen. It is called Phone-T.V.
>
> A third new machine is a TTY for the deaf-blind. The deaf-blind person can read it by running his hands over the raised print.
>
> Some stores have TTY's now. A deaf person can call the store to buy things. More important, some police stations have TTY's, too. Already lives have been saved.[3]

Another means of electronic stimulation in the treatment of sensori-neural hearing loss is also still in the experimental stages. This is a surgical procedure called cochlear implant. It involves implantation of small electrode arrays into the nerve fibers of the snail-shaped cochlea of the inner ear. An A.M. radio frequency system or an electromagnetic coupling transmits sound signals from an external device behind the ear to the internal receivers. By this means, patients are enabled to hear a broader range of frequencies at increased intensities.

The technique has not yet been refined to the point that it makes *understanding of speech* possible for the totally deaf, but future improvements may make that possibility a reality. In a paper presented at the May, 1975 meeting of the Royal Society of Medicine in London, R.P. Michelson, M.D., stated: "Our group have presently under design consideration an implantable device consisting of eight channels whereby the frequency elements of speech would be delivered to the appropriate 'frequency place' of the neaural array in the basal membrane."[4]

Even though cochlear implants cannot, at the present time, make speech understandable for the deaf, they do help in enhancing lip-reading skills and by creating awareness of environmental sounds. This surgical procedure is already making cracks in the wall that imprisons the deaf. Hopefully, it will not be too long before speech discrimination will also be made possible by this method, bringing about the collapse of the remainder of that wall.

These are only a few of the newer developments in the field of electronics that may help the hearing handicapped. More and better ones are sure to be on the way. But technology is not responsible for all of the new ideas. Ever hear of a hearing-ear dog? The American Humane Association is working on a training program for such animals. The program teaches dogs to bring certain sounds to the attention of their masters: a child crying, a doorbell, a car horn. Ruth Deschene, society director, says that the dogs catch on quickly and can be trained in six weeks.

In the medical field, one of many new developments involves the use of transplants, including eardrums and the small bones of the middle ear. The University of Cincinnati has instituted a nonprofit ear bank for such transplants. The parts can be ordered by mail and delivered directly to hospitals. Dr. S. George Lesinski, Director of the Division of Neurootology at the University of Cincinnati College of Medicine, said that he and his staff had performed eighteen transplants over the past year with ninety percent success. He emphasized, though, that the operation cannot help a person whose hearing loss results from nerve problems.

Research laboratories associated with medical schools and hearing centers throughout the United States are working to develop a better understanding of hearing problems and to devise new methods of treatment and rehabilitation. But they need more financial support! Public interest needs to be stimulated before this increased support will come about. Write to National Association of the Deaf to see what *you* can do.

Another hope for the future is that more health insurance companies will provide benefits for purposes of aural rehabilitation. A friend who had purchased a new hearing aid recently said to me, "Not many people can afford the luxury of being hard of hearing these days." Well, we hope that will change. Not only should the price of hearing aids be covered by a good policy, but so should continued therapy in lipreading, auditory training, and speech rehabilitation. When is the public going to wake up to the fact that these are not frills? They are very real needs, connected with the nation's most prevalent health problem—hearing loss.

What about acupuncture as a treatment for nerve deafness? News stories have told of acupuncture centers, mostly on the East and West Coasts, that have claimed success in treating nerve deafness. One report comes from Dr. Alfred Peng of New York's Saint Luke's Hospital. The study there involved ten people who had been deaf for five to thirty-one years. The report claimed that eight of the ten patients

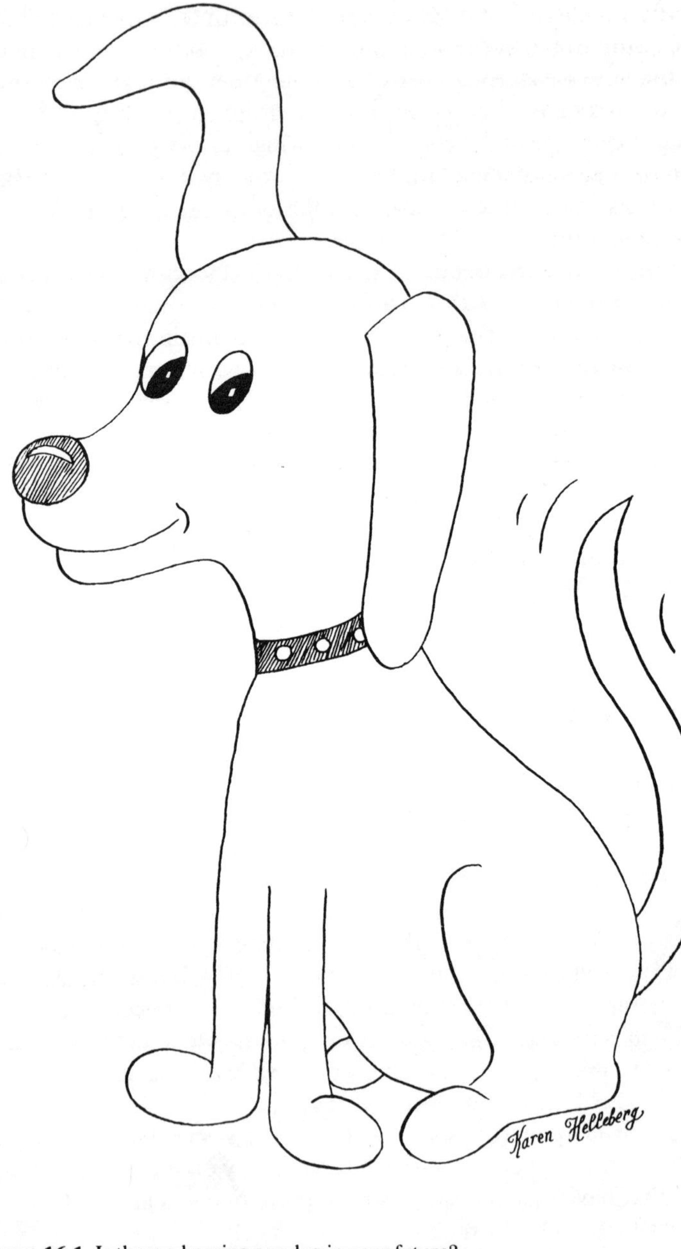

Figure 16.1. Is there a hearing ear dog in your future?

showed some degree of improvement.[5] According to its proponents, acupuncture can sometimes improve the function of nerve tissue made insensitive by strokes or degenerative diseases. *But,* let me warn you that work in this area is highly experimental. I think we should keep an open mind about any technique that shows some promise of helping the hearing impaired, but there just isn't enough solid evidence at this time to support the claims made for acupuncture as a treatment for sensori-neural hearing loss. Many American doctors are skeptical about it. In fact, the American Council of Otolaryngology has issued a statement that its research has not turned up evidence to support acupuncture therapy for hearing loss. So, unless and until there is more conclusive evidence, my advice to you is, wait and see.

The developments I've mentioned here are only a small sampling of the exciting things that are happening in the field of audiological research. Every year brings further advances. My hope for your future wears bright wings.

You and I have been together, now, through many pages. I hope I won't sound too sentimental when I say that, during the two years that I have been compiling and writing this book, I've come to think of you, not as some vague, faceless reader "out there," but as a friend. I hope I have given you some answers you've needed, and that you'll continue to use this book as a reference and guide. If I've given you nothing else, I'd at least like to believe that I leave with you the sure knowledge that someone cares very deeply about you and the problems you face.

Henry Ward Beecher said, "Every tomorrow has two handles. We can take hold of it with the handle of anxiety or the handle of faith."

Here's to your tomorrow, my friend!

Notes

Chapter 1

[1]Nanette Fabray, in Better Hearing Institute, *They Overcame Hearing Loss,* p. 4.

[2]McCay Vernon, "Fifty Years of Research on the Intelligence of the Deaf and Hard of Hearing: A Survey of the Literature and Discussion of Implications," *Journal of Rehabilitation of the Deaf* 2 (1968): 12.

[3]Larry Brown, in *They Overcame Hearing Loss,* p. 1.

[4]Tony Zale, in *They Overcame Hearing Loss,* p. 12.

[5]Vance Hartke, in *They Overcame Hearing Loss,* p. 5.

[6]Norm Crosby, in *They Overcame Hearing Loss,* p. 2.

[7]Dency Day, in *They Overcame Hearing Loss,* p. 3.

[8]Sol Lesser, in *They Overcame Hearing Loss,* p. 6.

[9]Frederic March, in *They Overcame Hearing Loss,* p. 7.

[10]Dale Milford, in *They Overcame Hearing Loss,* p. 8.

[11]Fred O'Green, in *They Overcame Hearing Loss,* p. 9.

[12]Johnnie Ray, in *They Overcame Hearing Loss,* p. 10.

[13]George C. Wallace, in *They Overcame Hearing Loss,* p. 11.

[14]U.S. Department of Health, Education, and Welfare, *Hearing Loss: Hope through Research,* p. 3.

Chapter 2

[1]This analogy is adapted, with the author's permission, from a similar one given by Hayes A. Newby, in *Audiology,* p. 7.

[2]Joseph R. Di Bartolomeo, "Anatomy and Physiology of the Ear," in *Introductory Hearing Science,* ed. Sanford E. Gerber, p. 11.

Chapter 3

[1]John Ballantyne, *Deafness,* p. 44.

[2]Ibid., p. 43.

[3]Norton Canfield, *Hearing: A Handbook for Laymen,* p. 123.

[4]Ibid., p. 100.

[5]Ibid., p. 62.

[6]Ibid., p. 101.

[7]Hallowell Davis, "Abnormal Hearing and Deafness," in *Hearing and Deafness,* ed. Hallowell Davis and S. Richard Silverman, p. 108.

Chapter 4

[1]John Ballantyne, *Deafness,* p. 147.

[2]I. Friedman, "The Pathology of Deafness," in *Sensorineural Hearing Loss,* ed. G. E. W. Wolstenholme, p. 56.

[3]Ballantyne, p. 152.

[4]Ibid., p. 154.

[5]Norton Canfield, *Hearing: A Handbook for Laymen,* p. 68.

[6]Hayes Newby, *Audiology,* p. 53.

[7]"Need to hear better? You Can!" *Changing Times: The Kiplinger Magazine,* August 1975, p. 29.

[8]Stephen Prescod, in a report released by Andrews University, Berrien Springs, Mich. (UPI, July 1975).

[9]Newby, p. 51.

[10]John F. Corso, "Age and Sex Differences in Pure-tone Thresholds," *A.M.A. Archives of Otolaryngology,* 77 (1963): 398-99.

[11]Canfield, p. 71.

Chapter 5

[1]Lynn Thorndike, *A History of Magic and Experimental Science* (New York: Columbia University Press, 1923), Vol. 2, pp. 561 and 145-46, cited by Hallowell Davis in *Hearing and Deafness,* ed. Hallowell Davis and S. Richard Silverman, 3rd ed. (New York: Holt, Rinehart and Winston, 1970), p. 3.

[2]John Ballantyne, *Deafness,* p. 112.

[3]Hayes A. Newby, *Audiology,* p. 43.

[4]Harold F. Schuknecht, "Stapedectomy Operation for Hearing Loss from Otosclerosis," *Sound* 1 (1962): 16-21.

[5]Newby, p. 21.

[6]David S. Akens, *Loss of Hearing and You,* p. 93.

[7]Herman G. Wallenfels, *Hearing Aids for Nerve Deafness,* p. 15.

[8]Newby, p. 56.

[9]Ross J. Roeser, John C. Campbell, and David D. Daly, "Recovery of Auditory Functions Following Meningitic Deafness," *Journal of Speech and Hearing Disorders* 40 ((1975): 405.[10]"Need to Hear Better? You Can!"
Changing Times: The Kiplinger Magazine, *August 1975, p. 27.*

Chapter 7

[1]"Need to Hear Better? You Can!" *Changing Times: The Kiplinger Magazine,* August 1975, p. 27.

[2]Derek A. Sanders, *Aural Rehabilitation,* p. 180.

[3]Hayes Newby, *Audiology,* p. 43.

[4]Ibid., p. 330.

[5]Herman G. Wallenfels, *Hearing Aids for Nerve Deafness,* p. vi.

[6]David S. Akens, *Loss of Hearing and You,* p. 57.

[7]S. R. Silverman and Hallowell Davis, "Counseling About Hearing Aids," in *Hearing and Deafness,* ed. Hallowell Davis and S. Richard Silverman, p. 322.

[8]Wallenfels, p. 102.

[9]Silverman and Davis, p. 318.

[10]"Need to Hear Better?" p. 28.

[11]Wallenfels, p. 62.

[12]*Facts about Hearing Aids,* p. 12. Reprinted with permission from Council of Better Business Bureaus, Inc.

[13]Sanders, p. 175.

[14]J. Jerger, R. Carhart, and D. Dirks, "Binaural Hearing Aids and Speech Intelligibility," *Journal of Speech and Hearing Research* 4: 147.

[15]Earl Harford and Joseph Barry, "A Rehabilitative Approach to the Problems of Unilateral Hearing Impairment: The Contralateral Routing of Signals (CROS)," *Journal of Speech and Hearing Disorders* 30 (1965): 121-38.

[16]Alfred R. Dunlavy, "CROS: The New Miracle Worker," *Audecibel* 19 (1970): 141-48.

[17]*Facts about Hearing Aids,* p. 7.

[18]"Need to Hear Better?" p. 28

[19]Bill Cosby, on "The Johnny Carson Show," 8 March 1976.

Chapter 8

[1]Some of the recommendations in this section are adapted from *Learning to Hear Again* by Sidney Blackstone. Reprinted from *Volta Review* with permission from the Alexander Graham Bell Association for the Deaf, Washington, D.C.

[2]Herman G. Wallenfels, *Hearing Aids for Nerve Deafness,* p. 44.

[3]Please see Chapter 12 for other suggestions that will help you to cope with your emotional reactions to your loss of hearing.

Chapter 9

[1]Mark Ross, *Principles of Aural Rehabilitation,* p. 31.

[2]Olive Wyatt, *Teach Yourself Lip-reading,* p. xix.

[3]Derek A. Sanders, *Aural Rehabilitation,* p. 295.

[4]Ibid., p. 87.

Chapter 10

[1]Raymond Carhart, "Auditory Training," in *Hearing and Deafness,* ed. Hallowell Davis and S. Richard Silverman, p. 373.

[2]Hayes A. Newby, *Audiology,* p. 365.

[3]Derek A. Sanders, *Aural Rehabilitation,* p. 227.

[4]J. C. Kelly, *Clinician's Handbook for Auditory Training,* p. 28. Reprinted with permission from the Alexander Graham Bell Association for the Deaf, Inc.

[5]Ibid., p. 5.

[6]Ibid., p. 39.

[7]Sanders, p. 272.

Chapter 11

[1]Hayes A. Newby, *Audiology,* p. 248.

[2]*Noise and You: The ABC's of Hearing Conservation,* p. 13.

[3]Ibid., p. 12.

[4]Walter L. Leonetti, "You Can't Reload Your Hearing," p. 63. Reprinted by permission from *The American Rifleman.* Further reproduction without permission is prohibited.

[5]W. Dixon Ward, "Effects of Noise on Hearing Thresholds," in *Noise as a Public Health Hazard,* ed. W. Dixon Ward and James E. Fricke, p. 44.

[6]*ABC's of Hearing Conservation,* p. 7.

[7]Ibid., p. 12.

[8]David M. Lipscomb, "Noise in the Environment: The Problem," in *Maico Audiological Library Series,* Vol. 8, p. 1.

[9]William F. Rintelmann, "A Review of Research Concerning Rock and Roll Music and Noise-induced Hearing Loss," in *Maico Audiological Library Series,* Vol. 8, p. 26.

[10]Maurice H. Miller, "Speech and Voice Patterns Associated with Hearing Impairment," in *Maico Audiological Library Series,* Vol. 2, p. 18.

[11]Philip E. Rosenberg, "Auditory Rehabilitation," in *Maico Audiological Library Series,* Vol. 1, p. 29.

[12]Raymond Carhart, "Development and Conservation of Speech," in *Hearing and Deafness,* ed. Hallowell Davis and S. Richard Silverman, p. 370.

[13]Newby, p. 346.

Chapter 12

[1]Joseph Sataloff, *Hearing Loss,* p. 342.

[2]D. A. Ramsdell, "The Psychology of the Hard-of-Hearing and The Deafened Adult," in *Hearing and Deafness,* ed. Hallowell Davis and S. Richard Silverman, p. 442.

[3]Kenneth M. Day, cited by John Ballantyne in *Deafness,* p. 247.

[4]Sataloff, p. 445.

[5]Ramsdell, pp. 436-42.

[6]Ibid., p. 437.

[7]Ibid., p. 439.

[8]Martin E. P. Seligman, "Fall into Helplessness," *Psychology Today,* June 1973, p. 43.

[19]Reprinted by permission from GUIDEPOSTS MAGAZINE, Copyright (1971) by Guideposts Associates, Inc., Carmel, New York 10512. August, 1971, pp. 22-24.

[10]Dan G. Pettingill, "Adjustments of the Deaf," in *Deaf Adults.*

[11]Frederick Schreiber, "Priority Needs," in *Deaf Adults.*

Chapter 13

[1]Anne Roe, *The Psychology of Occupations,* pp. 23-39.

[2]A. S. Lunde and S. G. Bigman, *Occupational Conditions among the Deaf.*

[3]*Skilled Eyes and Hands of the Deaf,* pp. 3-4.

[4]McCay Vernon, "Potential Achievement, and Rehabilitation in the Deaf Population," *Rehabilitation Literature* 31 (1970).

[5]Ted J. Holdt, "Job Development, Finding and Assessment for the Deaf Worker," *Journal of Rehabilitation of the Deaf,* Monograph Number 2 February 1970, p. 59.

[6]Earl T. Klein, "Employment Practices and Trends in Industry and Their Implications for the Deaf," *Journal of Rehabilitation of the Deaf,* Monograph Number 2 February 1970, p. 7.

[7]E. Ross Stuckless, cited by Robert R. Lauritsen, "An Effective Placement Program for Deaf Clients," *Journal of Rehabilitation of the Deaf,* Monograph Number 2 February 1970, p. 87.

[8]Klein, p. 7.

[9]Ibid., pp. 6-7.

[10]McCay Vernon and Judith Ann Snyder, "What's Available for Deaf People in Rehabilitation?" *ASHA, A Journal of the American Speech and Hearing Association* 14 (1972): pp. 51-56.

[11]G. Dewey Coats, cited by Lauritsen, pp. 79-80.

[12]William Williams, "Employment Practices and Trends in Large Industry," *Journal of Rehabilitation of the Deaf,* Monograph Number 2 February 1970, p. 16.

[13]Richard B. Sheridan, quoted in *The New Dictionary of Thoughts,* comp. Tryon Edwards (Standard Book Co., 1965), p. 645.

[14]Mervin Garretson, cited by Leo M. Jacobs in *A Deaf Adult Speaks Out* (Washington, D.C.: Galluadet College Press, 1974), p. 47.

[15]Margaret Kent, cited by Paul J. Ottinger in "Dr. David Denton: Total Communication," *The Deaf American,* October 1971, pp. 3-6.

[16]Vernon, "Potential Achievement," p. 2.

[17]Helen Keller, quoted in *The New Dictionary of Thoughts,* comp. Tryon Edwards (Standard Book Co., 1965), p. 646.

Chapter 14

[1]Joseph J. Rizzo, "Foreword" in *They Overcame Hearing Loss.*

[2]The April issue sells for $5.00 and can be ordered by writing to *American Annals of the Deaf,* 5034 Wisconsin Avenue, N.W., Washington, D.C. 20016.

Chapter 15

[1]Mildred Kennedy and Mary Wood Whitehurst, *Suggestions for Friends and Relatives of the Hard of Hearing,* p. 2. Reprinted by permission from The Alexander Graham Bell Association for the Deaf, Inc.

[2]Ibid., p. 4.

[3]Ibid., p. 5.

[4]Ibid., p. 4.

[5]Ibid., p. 1.

Chapter 16

[1]Norton Canfield, *Hearing: A Handbook for Laymen,* p. 210.

[2]Glen P. McCormick, "Wanted: 400 Who Otherwise Might Never

Talk," *West Virginia University Magazine,* Fall, 1972, pp. 2-7.

[3]Lee Brody, "Deaf People and TTY's," in *I'm Deaf Too: 12 Deaf Americans,* p. 14.

[4]R. P. Michelson, "Cochlear Implants," *Journal of Laryngology and Otology* 90 (1976), p. 444.

[5]Alfred Peng, quoted in *Newsweek,* 12 March 1973, p. 32.

Bibliography

Akens, David S. *Loss of Hearing and You.* Huntsville, Ala.: Strode, 1970.

Ballantyne, John. *Deafness.* 2nd ed. London: J. & A. Churchill, 1970.

Barker, Roger G.; Wright, Beatrice A.; Meyerson, Lee; Gonick, Mollie R. *Adjustments to Physical Handicap and Illness: A Survey of Physique and Disability.* Rev. ed. New York: Social Science Research Council, 1953.

Baron, Robert Alexander. *The Tyranny of Noise.* New York: St. Mary's Press, 1970.

Better Hearing Institute: *They Overcame Hearing Loss.* Washington, D.C.: Better Hearing Institute, 1973.

Blackstone, Sidney. *Learning to Hear Again.* Volta Bureau Reprint No. 565. Washington, D.C.: Volta Bureau, n. d.

Bolton, Brian, Cull, John G., and Hardy, Richard E. "Psychological Adjustment to Hearing Loss and Deafness." In *Educational and Psychosocial Aspects of Deafness,* edited by Richard E. Hardy and John G. Cull. Springfield, Ill.: Charles C. Thomas, 1970.

Bowe, Frank, and Sternberg, Martin. *I'm Deaf Too: 12 Deaf Americans.* Silver Spring, Md.: National Association of the Deaf, 1973.

Bradley, Wesley J., M. D. "How Modern Life Can Damage Your Hearing." *U.S. News & World Report,* 3 May 1976, pp. 57, 60.

Brody, Lee. "Deaf People and TTY'S." In *I'm Deaf Too: 12 Deaf Americans.* Silver Spring, Md.: National Association of the Deaf, 1973.

Burns, William. *Noise and Man.* Philadelphia: J. B. Lippincott, 1969.

Canfield, Norton. *Hearing: A Handbook for Laymen.* Garden City, N.Y.: Doubleday, 1959.

Carhart, Raymond. "Auditory Training." In *Hearing and Deafness,* edited by Hallowell Davis and S. Richard Silverman. Rev. ed. New York: Holt, Rinehart, and Winston, 1965.

———"Development and Conservation of Speech." In *Hearing and Deaf-*

ness, edited by Hallowell Davis and S. Richard Silverman. 3rd ed. New York: Holt, Rinehart, and Winston, 1970.

Corso, John F. "Age and Sex Differences in Puretone Thresholds." *A.M.A. Archives of Otolaryngology* 77 (1963): 398-99.

———"Proposed Laboratory Standard of Normal Hearing." In *Hearing Measurement: A Book of Readings,* edited by Ira M. Ventry, Joseph B. Chaiklin, and Richard F. Dixon. New York: Appleton-Century-Crofts, 1971.

Council Membership Directory. Washington, D.C.: Council of Organizations Serving the Deaf, 1974.

Craig, William N., and Craig, Helen B., eds. "Programs and Services for the Deaf in the United States." *American Annals of the Deaf* 122 (1977).

Craig, William N., and Silver, N. H. "Examination of Selected Employment Problems of the Deaf." *American Annals of the Deaf,* 1962.

Crammatte, A. B. "The Adult-Deaf in Professions." *American Annals of the Deaf,* 1962.

Davis, Hallowell. "Abnormal Hearing and Deafness." In *Hearing and Deafness,* edited by Hallowell Davis and S. Richard Silverman. 3rd ed. New York: Holt, Rinehart, and Winston, 1970.

———"Acoustics and Psychoacoustics." In *Hearing and Deafness,* edited by Hallowell Davis and S. Richard Silverman. 3rd ed. New York: Holt, Rinehart and Winston, 1970.

———"Anatomy and Physiology of the Auditory System." In *Hearing and Deafness,* edited by Hallowell Davis and S. Richard Silverman. 3rd ed. New York: Holt, Rinehart and Winston, 1970.

———"Audiometry." In *Hearing and Deafness,* edited by Hallowell Davis and S. Richard Silverman. 3rd ed. New York: Holt, Rinehart and Winston, 1970.

Davis, Hallowell, and Fowler, E. P. "The Medical Treatment of Hearing Loss and the Conversation of Hearing." In *Hearing and Deafness,* edited by Hallowell Davis and S. Richard Silverman. 3rd ed. New York: Holt, Rinehart and Winston, 1970.

Dunlavy, Alfred R. "CROS: The New Miracle Worker." *Audecibel* 29 (1970).

Ewing, Sir Alexander, and Ewing, Lady Ethel C. *Hearing Aids, Lipreading and Clear Speech.* Manchester, England: Manchester University Press, 1967.

Facts About Hearing Aids. Washington, D.C.: Council of Better Business Bureaus, Inc., 1973.

Fowler, Edmund Prince, Sr. *Twenty Years of Research in Otosclerosis, and Correlated Problems, 1926–1946.* New York: Central Bureau of Research, American Otological Society, 1946.

Friedman, I. "The Pathology of Deafness." In *Sensorineural Hearing Loss,* edited by G. E. W. Wolstenholme and Julie Knight. London: The Ciba Foundation, J. & A. Churchill, 1970.

Gerber, Sanford E. *Introductory Hearing Science: Physical and Psychological Concepts.* Philadelphia: W. B. Saunders Company, 1974.

Goodhill, V. "Pathology, Diagnosis and Therapy of Deafness." In *Hand-*

book of Speech Pathology, edited by L. E. Travis. New York: Appleton-Century-Crofts, 1957.

Gowan, John C. "Guidance of the Deaf." In *Persons with Hearing Loss,* edited by Jerry Griffith. Springfield, Ill.: Charles C. Thomas, 1969.

Griffith, Jerry. *Persons with Hearing Loss.* Springfield, Ill.: Charles C. Thomas, 1969.

Hardy, Miriam Pauls. "Speechreading." In *Hearing and Deafness,* edited by Hallowell Davis and S. Richard Silverman. 3rd ed. New York: Holt, Rinehart and Winston, 1970.

Hardy, Richard E., and Cull, John G. *Educational and Psychosocial Aspects of Deafness.* Springfield, Ill.: Charles C. Thomas, 1974.

Harford, Earl, and Barry, Joseph. "A Rehabilitative Approach to the Problem of Unilateral Hearing Impairment: The Contralateral Routing of Signals (CROS)." *Journal of Speech and Hearing Disorders* 30 (1965): 121-38.

Hartbauer, R. D. *Aural Habilitation.* Springfield, Ill.: Charles C. Thomas, 1975.

Haspiel, George S. *A Synthetic Approach to Lip Reading.* Magnolia, Mass.: Expression Company, 1964.

"Hearing Aids and the Older American." *The Volta Review,* November 1973, pp. 464-66.

Helleberg, Marilyn. "How to Aim Yourself." *Guideposts,* August 1971, pp. 22-24.

Hirsch, Ira J. "Auditory Training." In *Hearing and Deafness,* edited by Hallowell Davis and S. Richard Silverman. 3rd ed. New York: Holt, Rinehart, and Winston, 1970.

———"Recent Development in Hearing-Aid Use." *Round Table on Hearing Aids.* International Audiology 5 (1966).

Hochberg, Irving. *Interpretation of Audiometric Results.* Indianapolis: Bobbs-Merrill, 1973.

Holdt, Ted J. "Implications of Technological Changes for Employment of Deaf Persons." *Journal of Rehabilitation of the Deaf,* Monograph Number 2, February 1970, pp. 63-73.

Hoops, Richard A. "Assessment and Evaluation: Differential Diagnosis of Hearing Loss." In *Persons with Hearing Loss,* edited by Jerry Griffith. Springfield, Ill.: Charles C. Thomas, 1969.

Hopkins, L. A., and Macklin, M. T. "Studies on the Inheritance of Deafness in the Pupils of the Clarke School for the Deaf." *The Laryngoscope* 56 (1946): 570-601.

Hudgins, C. V. "Auditory Training: Its Possibilities and Limitations." *Volta Review* 56 (1954): 1.

Hunt, Joseph. "State-federal Vocational Rehabilitation Program." *Vocational Rehabilitation of Deaf Persons.* U.S. Department of Health, Education and Welfare, 1968.

Hutton, Charles L., Jr. "Aural Rehabilitation." In *Persons with Hearing Loss,* edited by Jerry Griffith. Springfield, Ill.: Charles C. Thomas, 1969.

Jacobs, Leo M. *A Deaf Adult Speaks Out.* Washington, D.C.: Gallaudet College Press, 1974.

Jerger, James F.; Carhart, Raymond; Tillman, Tom W.; and Peterson, John L. "Some Relations Between Normal Hearing for Pure Tones and for Speech." In *Hearing Measurement: A Book of Readings,* edited by Ira M. Ventry, Joseph B. Chaiklin and Richard F. Dixon. New York: Appleton-Century-Crofts, 1971.

Jerger, J., Carhart, R., and Dirks, D. "Binaural Hearing Aids and Speech Intelligibility." *Journal of Speech and Hearing Research* 4 (1961): 137-48.

Kelly, J. C. *Clinician's Handbook for Auditory Training.* Washington, D.C.: The Alexander Graham Bell Association for the Deaf, 1953.

Kennedy, Mildred, and Whitehurst, Mary Wood. *Suggestions for Friends and Relatives of the Hard of Hearing.* Washington, D.C.: The Alexander Graham Bell Association for the Deaf, 1969.

Klein, Earl T. "Employment Practices and Trends in Large Industry." *Journal of Rehabilitation of the Deaf,* Monograph Number 2, February 1970, pp. 15-21.

Knapp, P. H. "Emotional Aspects of Hearing Loss." *Psychosomatic Medicine* 10 (1948): 203-22.

Kronenberg, H. H., and Blake, G. D. *Young Deaf Adults: An Occupational Survey.* U.S. Department of Health, Education and Welfare, 1965.

Kryter, Karl D. *The Effects of Noise on Man.* New York: Academic Press, 1970.

Lauritsen, Robert R. "New Vistas for Competitive Employment of Deaf Persons." *Journal of Rehabilitation of the Deaf,* Monograph Number 2, February 1970, pp. 92-100.

Lederer, Francis L., and Hollender, Abraham R. *Textbook of the Ear, Nose, and Throat.* Philadelphia: Davis, 1947.

Leonetti, Walter L. "You Can't Reload Your Hearing." *The American Rifleman,* September 1972, pp. 62-64.

Leszcanski, Lidia. "Device for Feeling Vibrations Is Helping the Deaf to 'Hear'." *Omaha World Herald* 12 May 1974, p. 13-A.

Lewis, Arthur H. "World's Safest Drivers." *Ford Times,* March 1948, pp. 6-8.

Lipscomb, David M. "Noise in the Environment: The Problem." *Maico Audiological Library Series.* Vol. 8. Maico Hearing Instruments, 1970.

Lowell, E. L. *Higher Education for the Deaf.* Edited by D. Cutler, U.S. Department of Health, Education and Welfare, 1965.

Lunde, A. S., and Bigman, S. G. *Occupational Conditions Among the Deaf.* Washington, D.C.: Gallaudet College Press, 1959.

McCormick, Glen P. "Wanted: 400 Who Otherwise Might Never Talk," *West Virginia University Magazine,* Fall, 1972, pp. 2-7.

Martin, N. A. "Psychogenic Deafness." *Annals of Otolaryngology, Rhinology, and Laryngology* 55 (1946): 81-89.

Mayer, Lyle V. *Fundamentals of Voice and Diction.* Rev. ed. Dubuque, Iowa: William C. Brown, 1968.

Michelson, R. P., M.D. "Cochlear Implants," *Journal of Laryngology and Otology* 90 (1976), pp. 441-44.

Miller, Maurice H. *Hearing Aids.* Indianapolis: Bobbs-Merrill, 1972.

———"Speech and Voice Patterns Associated with Hearing Impairment."

In *Maico Audiological Library Series.* Vol. 2. Maico Hearing Instruments, 1967.

Montague, Harriet. *Lip Reading Lessons for Adult Beginners.* Washington, D.C.: Volta Bureau, 1945.

Myklebust, H. R. *The Psychology of Deafness.* Rev. ed. New York: Grune and Stratton, 1964.

"Need to hear better? You can!" *Changing Times: The Kiplinger Magazine,* August, 1975, pp. 27-30.

Nemoy, Elizabeth McGenly, and Davis, Serena Foley. *The Correction of Defective Consonant Sounds.* Boston: Expression, 1937.

Newby, Hayes A. *Audiology.* 3rd ed. New York: Appleton-Century-Crofts, 1972.

Noise and You: The ABC's of Hearing Conservation. Greenfield, Mass.: Channing L. Bete, 1970.

Olson, Ann. *Educating the Deaf.* Unpublished paper, 1975.

O'Neill, John J., and Oyer, Herbert J. *Visual Communication for the Hard of Hearing.* Englewood Cliffs, N.J.: Prentice-Hall, 1961.

Ordman, Kathryn A., and Ralli, Mary P. *What People Say.* New York: The Nitchie School of Lip Reading, 1949.

Ottinger, Paul J. "Dr. David Denton: Total Communication." *The Deaf American,* October 1971, pp. 3-6.

Oyer, Herbert J. *Auditory Communication for the Hard of Hearing.* Englewood Cliffs, N.J.: Prentice-Hall, 1961.

Peng, Alfred. Item in *Newsweek,* 12 March 1973.

Pettingill, Don G. "Adjustments of the Deaf." In *Deaf Adults.* Silver Spring, Md.: National Association of the Deaf, 1964.

Pool, J. Lawrence, and Pava, Arthur A. *Acoustic Nerve Tumors.* Springfield, Ill.: Charles C. Thomas, 1957.

Prescod, Stephen. Report released by Andrews University, Berrien Springs, Michigan. UPI, July 1975.

Ramsdell, D. A. "The Psychology of the Hard-of-Hearing and the Deafened Adult." In *Hearing and Deafness,* edited by Hallowell Davis and S. Richard Silverman. 3rd ed. New York: Holt, Rinehart, and Winston, 1970.

Reed, Sheldon. *Counseling and Medical Genetics.* Philadelphia: Saunders, 1963.

Rintelmann, William F. "A Review of Research Concerning Rock and Roll Music and Noise-induced Hearing Loss." In *Maico Audiological Library Series.* Vol. 8. Maico Hearing Instruments, 1970.

Roe, Anne. *The Psychology of Occupations.* New York: Wiley, 1956.

Roeser, Ross J., Campbell, John C., and Daly, David D. "Recovery of Auditory Function Following Meningitic Deafness." *Journal of Speech and Hearing Disorders* 40 (1975): 405-11.

Rosen, S. "Simple Method for Restoring Hearing in Otosclerosis: Mobilization of the Stapes." *Acta Oto-Laryngologica* 44 (1954): 78-88.

Rosenberg, Philip E. "Auditory Rehabilitation." In *Maico Audiological Library Series.* Vol. 1. Maico Hearing Instruments, 1967.

Ross, Mark. *Principles of Aural Rehabilitation.* Indianapolis: Bobbs-Merrill, 1972.

Sanders, Derek A. *Aural Rehabilitation.* Englewood Cliffs, N.J.: Prentice-Hall, 1971.

Sanders, Jay W., and Rintelmann, William F. "Masking in Audiometry." In *Hearing Measurement: A Book of Readings,* edited by Ira M. Ventry, Joseph B. Chaiklin and Richard F. Dixon. New York: Appleton-Century-Crofts, 1971.

Sataloff, Joseph. *Hearing Loss.* Philadelphia: J. B. Lippincott, 1966.

Savisaari, Runo. "Compensating for Severe Undertraining." *Vocational Rehabilitation of Deaf Persons.* U.S. Department of Health, Education, and Welfare, 1968.

Schein, J. D., and Bushnaq, S. "Higher Education for the Deaf in the United States: A Retrospective Investigation." *American Annals of the Deaf,* 1972.

Schreiber, Frederick C. "The Deaf Adult's Point of View." *Deaf Adults.* Silver Spring, Md.: National Association of the Deaf, 1971.

———"Priority Needs." *Deaf Adults.* Silver Spring, Md.: National Association of the Deaf, 1971.

Schuknecht, Harold F., ed. *Otosclerosis.* Boston: Little, Brown, 1962.

Seigenthaler, Bruce M. "Audiogram-Average Methods and SRT Scores." In *Hearing Measurement: A Book of Readings,* edited by Ira M. Ventry, Joseph B. Chaiklin and Richard F. Dixon. New York: Appleton-Century-Crofts, 1971.

Seligman, Martin E. P. "Fall into Helplessness." *Psychology Today,* June 1973, pp. 43-48.

Senturia, B. H. *Diseases of the External Ear.* Springfield, Ill.: Charles C. Thomas, 1957.

Silverman, S. Richard, and Davis, Hallowell. "Counseling About Hearing Aids." In *Hearing and Deafness,* edited by Hallowell Davis and S. Richard Silverman. 3rd ed. New York: Holt, Rinehart, and Winston, 1970.

Silverman, S. Richard, and Taylor, S. Gordon. "The Choice and Use of Hearing Aids." In *Hearing and Deafness,* edited by Hallowell Davis and S. Richard Silverman. Rev. ed. New York: Holt, Rinehart and Winston, 1965.

Skilled Eyes and Hands of the Deaf. Lansing: Michigan Employment Security Commission, 1968.

Switzer, Mary E., and Williams, Boyce R. "Life Problems of Deaf People." In *Deaf Adults.* Silver Spring, Md.: National Association of the Deaf, 1971.

U.S. Department of Health, Education, and Welfare, *Hearing Loss: Hope through Research,* Washington, D.C.: Health Information Series, No. 53, pp. 3-30.

Van Egmond, A. A. J. "Congenital Deafness." *Journal of Laryngology and Otology* 68 (1954): 429-43.

Van Riper, Charles. *Speech Correction: Principles and Methods.* 5th ed. Englewood Cliffs, N.J.: Prentice-Hall, 1972.

Vernon, McCay. "Available Training Opportunities for Deaf People." In *Rehabilitation Literature.* Silver Spring, Md.: National Association of the Deaf.

———"Fifty Years of Research on the Intelligence of the Deaf and Hard of Hearing: A Survey of the Literature and Discussion of Implications." *Journal of Rehabilitation of the Deaf* 2 (1968): 1-12.

———"Potential Achievement, and Rehabilitation in the Deaf Population." In *Rehabilitation Literature.* Chicago: National Easter Seal Society for Crippled Children and Adults, September, 1970.

———"Sociological and Psychological Factors Associated with Hearing Loss." *Journal of Speech and Hearing Research* 12 (1969): 541-63.

Vernon, McCay, and Makowsky, Bernard. "Deafness and Minority Group Dynamics." *The Deaf Americans* 21 (1969): 2-6.

Vernon, McCay, and Snyder, Judith Ann. "What's Available for Deaf People in Rehabilitation?" *ASHA, A Journal of the American Speech and Hearing Association* 14 (1972): pp. 51-57.

Victoreen, J. A. *Hearing Enhancement.* Springfield, Ill.: Charles C. Thomas, 1960.

Wallenfels, Herman G. *Hearing Aids for Nerve Deafness.* Springfield, Ill.: Charles C. Thomas, 1971.

Walsh, T. E. "The Surgical Treatment of Hearing Loss." In *Hearing and Deafness,* edited by Hallowell Davis, and S. Richard Silverman. 3rd ed. New York: Holt, Rinehart and Winston, 1970.

Ward, W. Dixon. "Effects of Noise on Hearing Thresholds." In *Noise as a Public Health Hazard,* edited by W. Dixon Ward and James E. Fricke. American Speech and Hearing Association Journal (ASHA) Report 4. Washington, D.C.: The American Speech and Hearing Association, 1969.

West, Robert, and Ansberry, Merle. *The Rehabilitation of Speech.* New York: Harper and Row, 1968.

Whitehurst, Mary W. *Train Your Hearing.* Washington, D.C.: Volta Bureau, 1947.

Whitehurst, Mary W., and Monsees, Edna K. *Auditory Training for the Deaf.* Washington, D.C.: Volta Bureau, 1952.

Williams, Boyce R., and Vernon, McCay. "Vocational Guidance for the Deaf." In *Hearing and Deafness,* edited by Hallowell Davis and S. Richard Silverman. 3rd ed. New York: Holt, Rinehart, and Winston, 1970.

Williams, William. "Employment Practices and Trends: A Discussion." *Journal of Rehabilitation of the Deaf,* February 1970, pp. 22-24.

Wyatt, Olive M. *Teach Yourself Lip-reading.* Springfield, Ill.: Charles C. Thomas, 1969.

Index